Guidelines for Designing Usable Health Information Systems

Dedication

I dedicate this book to my esteemed mentors, particularly the visionary healthcare technology leader whose pioneering insights into digital transformation have profoundly shaped my understanding of the industry, my valued colleagues, whose wisdom, guidance, and unwavering support have been instrumental in shaping both my professional journey and the insights contained within these pages. Their expertise, encouragement, and collaborative spirit have not only inspired me to pursue this writing endeavour but have also enriched the knowledge and perspectives I am privileged to share. This work stands as a testament to the profound impact of their mentorship and the invaluable contributions they have made to my growth as both a practitioner and author.

I invite you to continue this journey with me and discover more insights and be a part of the ongoing conversation at
https://permaintegratedhealth.com/about-us/

You may reach me at **editor@permaintegratedhealth.com**

About the Author

Radhika Narayan – Founder, PERMA Integrated Health

I am a highly motivated Health IT professional with over 25 years of experience across the life sciences and healthcare sectors, including roles as Business Analyst, Product Owner, and Functional Product Trials & Beta Testing.

Currently, I am engaged in cutting-edge research examining how the 'Meaning' component of the PERMA model influences healthcare technology developers and their work outcomes. This research aims to uncover how a sense of purpose can enhance both personal satisfaction and professional effectiveness within the field of health technology.

Passionate about integrating positive psychology principles into practical applications, I am committed to advancing the standard of wellness through innovative solutions and evidence-based insights with the support of our community on this site.

Through PERMA Integrated Health, I share evidence-based insights, research, and practical guidance to help healthcare technology developers, care providers and organizations enhance engagement, wellness, and outcomes.

Table of Contents

Introduction.. 1

Chapter 01: Typical UI Mistakes in Health Information Systems & How to Avoid Them.. 4

    1. Cluttered Interfaces.. 4

    2. Inconsistent Visual Design...5

    3. Poor Navigation Structure..6

    4. Lack of Responsive Design..6

    5. Ignoring User Feedback..7

    6. Poor Data Visualization... 8

    7. Lack of Error Prevention and Feedback.............................. 8

    8. Overcomplicated Forms...9

    9. Inadequate Accessibility...10

    Conclusion...10

Chapter 02: Guidelines for UX Design in Health Information Systems: Principles, Practices, and Pitfalls.. 12

    1. Involve the User... 12

        Key Stages for Involving Users:.. 13

        Understanding the Diversity of Users:...........................14

        Use Case Scenario:..14

    2. Anticipate the User's Needs.. 15

        Key Considerations for Anticipating User Needs:.........15

        Use Case Scenario:.. 16

    3. Anticipate the User's Needs.. 17

    4. Maintain Consistency in Design... 19

        Key Considerations for Maintaining Consistency:........ 19

Use Case Scenario:... 20

5. Design Explorable Interfaces to Increase User Efficiency............ 21

Key Considerations for Designing Explorable Interfaces:............ 21

Use Case Scenario:... 22

6. Create Designs Which Help Users Minimize, Identify, and Rectify Errors.. 23

7. Protect the User's Work and Provide a Provision to Track the Status of Work... 24

8. Provide Visible Navigation...................................... 25

9. Train the End User.. 27

Do's and Don'ts of UX Design for HIS..............................28

References:...33

Chapter 03: Guidelines for GUI Design in Health Information Systems: Usability, Workflow, and Patient Safety.............................34

1. User-Centred Design (UCD) is Foundational......................35

2. Support Cognitive Workflows, Not Just Data Entry............... 37

3. Ensure Information is Accessible and Actionable.................39

4. Design for Safety and Error Prevention......................... 42

5. Follow Consistency and Standards...............................43

6. Design for Time-Critical Tasks................................. 45

7. Accommodate a Variety of User Expertise........................ 47

8. Incorporate Feedback and Iteration............................. 49

9. Support Interoperability and Integration....................... 51

10. Design for Privacy, Security, and Compliance.................. 53

Conclusion... 55

References:...57

Chapter 04: Do's and Don'ts of UX Design for Healthcare Information Systems...59

Do's...59

Don'ts...62

Putting People First...69

The Role of Communication and Collaboration......................69

The Importance of Simplicity and Clarity...............................70

Designing for Resilience...71

Ethics and Responsibility...71

Looking Ahead: Innovation and Opportunity.........................72

Final Thoughts..72

Chapter 05: Scientific Methods of UX Design........................74

Traditional UX Design: A Limited Approach............................74

Comparing Different Methods of Software Development Methodologies...75

Final Thoughts..77

Summary:...79

References:...79

Chapter 6: Does Quality Patient Care Ultimately Rely On Efficiently Designed HIS Interfaces?...80

Chapter 7: Few Myths and Realities of Health IT Systems.....................86

Chapter 8: Security -Privacy concerns and Usable HIS........................89

What is Security in Healthcare?...89

What is Privacy in Healthcare?..90

HIPAA privacy rules...94

Security with effective GUI; Use case scenarios:.....................96

References...105

Chapter 9: Positive Psychology and UX Design.................................. 106

   Usability and Its Importance in Digital Health Technologies.......... 108

      What is Usability?... 110

      Hypothetical Case Studies: Usability Nightmares in Health IT... 111

   Reflecting on the Consequences of Bad Usability.......................... 111

   Conclusion... 112

   References:..113

Chapter 10: Customer Journey Maps...115

   Customer Journey Maps (CJM):... 115

   My understanding:...117

   References:..117

Chapter 11: Final Thoughts – Designing Healthcare Information Systems (HIS) That Evolve with Care..119

   Key Takeaways from This eBook..119

A Call to Action... 122

Closing Note..123

Glossary:...124

Definitions:...129

References:...131

Preface

Given the growing reliance on digital systems in healthcare, the need for intuitive, efficient, and user-centred Health Information Systems (HIS) has never been more critical. These systems form the digital backbone of modern healthcare delivery, influencing everything from clinical decision-making to patient safety. Yet, despite their importance, many HIS interfaces remain complex and unintuitive, hindering rather than helping those who rely on them daily. This eBook, Guidelines for Designing Usable Screens for HIS, seeks to address this gap by offering practical insights, strategies, and best practices to support designers, developers, and healthcare professionals in creating systems that truly serve their users — and, ultimately, optimise healthcare workflows.

Purpose of this eBook

The primary purpose of this eBook is to offer clear, actionable guidelines for designing screens that are functional and user-friendly within Health Information Systems By focusing on usability, this guide seeks to improve the interaction between healthcare professionals and digital systems, ultimately contributing to improved patient care, operational efficiency, and user satisfaction. Whether you are designing interfaces for electronic health records (EHR), patient portals, or administrative tools, this eBook will equip you with the knowledge to create screens that are intuitive, accessible, and efficient.

The ultimate purpose of this eBook is to enable readers:

1. Reflect upon their common mistakes while designing graphical user interfaces for Health Information Systems

2. Follow common guidelines for designing effective Health Information Systems

3. Understand and ponder on how effective designs could enhance patient safety and address concerns about patient confidentiality and the security of health records.

4. Reflect on the Myths and realities of designing UI for Health Information Systems

5. Recognise why good designs are essential for Health Information Systems

Structure of this eBook

This eBook is structured to provide a comprehensive yet digestible approach to the topic. It begins with an introduction to the key principles of user interface design and usability, followed by detailed guidelines on layout, navigation, and visual hierarchy. The book then dives into the specifics of designing for different healthcare contexts, such as clinical, administrative, and mobile settings. Each chapter provides practical examples, common pitfalls, and suggestions for improvement, ensuring that readers not only understand the theory behind good design but also can apply it in their work. The final section offers insights into user testing and iterative design, highlighting the importance of feedback in refining HIS interfaces.

Target Audience for this eBook

This eBook is intended for a wide range of professionals involved in the design, development, and implementation of Health Information Systems It is particularly useful for UX/UI designers, product managers, developers, and healthcare IT specialists who seek to enhance the usability of HIS screens. Additionally, this guide is valuable for healthcare providers, administrators, and anyone interested in improving the digital experience within healthcare settings. By providing practical advice in a user-centred manner, this eBook ensures that everyone involved in the HIS design process can contribute to the creation of better, more usable systems

In summary, *Guidelines for Designing Usable Screens for HIS* is both a resource and a roadmap for creating user-centred, efficient, and effective Health Information Systems We hope that it serves as a valuable tool in your efforts to shape the future of healthcare technology.

Introduction

Within the contemporary healthcare ecosystem, Health Information Systems (HIS) play a critical role in improving patient care, enhancing operational efficiency, and streamlining administrative processes. As healthcare continues to embrace digital transformation, the design of these systems becomes more crucial than ever. However, while the technological advancements behind HIS are impressive, the usability of these systems often lags, impacting the effectiveness of healthcare delivery.

One of the most significant factors in determining how well HIS are adopted and utilised is the design of the screens that healthcare professionals interact with. Whether it's a nurse accessing patient records, a doctor recording diagnosis information, or an administrator managing appointments, the user interface plays a pivotal role in ensuring that the system is not only functional but also intuitive and easy to use. Poorly designed screens can lead to frustration, errors, and inefficiencies that ultimately compromise patient safety and care quality.

The goal of this book, *Guidelines for Designing Usable Health Information Systems*, is to provide practical guidance and expert insights into creating interfaces that prioritise usability without sacrificing functionality. This book takes a user-centred approach to screen design, emphasising the importance of designing with the needs of healthcare professionals in mind. By understanding the unique challenges faced by users in healthcare environments, we can create screens that enhance workflow, reduce cognitive load, and improve the overall user experience.

This book is not just for designers; it is for anyone involved in the creation or improvement of HIS, including developers, product managers, and healthcare professionals who interact with these systems daily. The guidelines and best practices outlined here are grounded in both theory and real-world experience, offering actionable advice that can be applied to any stage of the design process.

In the following chapters, we will explore fundamental design principles, such as information organisation, visual hierarchy, and interaction design, all tailored specifically for healthcare settings. We will discuss common challenges such as balancing complex data with simplicity, ensuring accessibility for diverse users, and maintaining a seamless user experience across various devices and platforms. Additionally, we will examine the importance of iterative testing and feedback, as well as how to continually refine and improve HIS interfaces.

Whether you're embarking on a new HIS design project or looking to optimise an existing system, this *e-book* will equip you with the tools and knowledge to make informed decisions and create interfaces that work for both healthcare professionals and patients. By prioritising usability in HIS design, we can not only improve the user experience but ultimately contribute to better patient outcomes and a more efficient healthcare system.

Chapter 01: Typical UI Mistakes in Health Information Systems & How to Avoid Them

When designing user interfaces for Health Information Systems (HIS), even small mistakes can have a significant impact on usability, efficiency, and, ultimately, patient care. Healthcare professionals depend on these systems to make critical decisions, manage complex data, and ensure seamless workflows. A poorly designed interface can slow down their tasks, create confusion, and even result in errors that could compromise patient safety.

In this chapter, we'll explore some of the most common UI mistakes made in HIS design and discuss strategies for avoiding them. By understanding and addressing these pitfalls, designers, and developers can create more effective, user-friendly screens that meet the needs of healthcare professionals and improve system performance.

1. Cluttered Interfaces

Mistake: Overloading a screen with too much information or too many options can overwhelm users, making it difficult for them to quickly identify what they need. Cluttered interfaces force users to scan the entire screen for relevant data, increasing cognitive load and the chances of errors.

Solution: Prioritise clarity and simplicity by focusing on the most essential information for the user's task at hand. Use white space effectively to separate distinct sections of the screen and avoid overwhelming the user with too many elements. Group related items together and utilise collapsible menus or tabs to organise information without overwhelming the display.

2. Inconsistent Visual Design

Mistake: Inconsistent design elements across screens or sections of the HIS can confuse users and create a fragmented experience. For instance, varying button styles, inconsistent colour schemes, or mixed typography can distract users and make navigation more difficult.

Solution: Establish a consistent design system for the entire HIS, including colour palettes, fonts, button styles, and icons. Consistent visual elements help users feel familiar with the interface, reducing their cognitive load and making it easier to navigate. Use standardised components like buttons, checkboxes, and dropdowns in a way that feels cohesive across the system.

3. Poor Navigation Structure

Mistake: One of the most frustrating issues in HIS design is a confusing or inefficient navigation structure. Users often have to click through multiple screens to find the information they need, or they may struggle with poorly organised menu items and labels. This not only wastes time but can also lead to users abandoning tasks or making mistakes in data entry.

Solution: Ensure that navigation is intuitive and consistent. Use a clear and logical hierarchy for menus and submenus. Group related items together and consider using breadcrumbs or navigation aids that show users where they are within the system. Always provide a 'back' button or a way to return to previous pages without losing data. Incorporate search functionality for quick access to commonly used features or records.

4. Lack of Responsive Design

Mistake: HIS interfaces that are not responsive can be especially problematic in today's diverse technological landscape. A screen that doesn't adapt properly to different device sizes or orientations can make it difficult for users to interact with the system, particularly in mobile or tablet environments, which are increasingly used in healthcare settings.

Solution: Design interfaces with responsiveness in mind, ensuring that the system works well on different devices (desktops, tablets, and smartphones) and screen sizes. Use a flexible layout that adapts to changes in screen size and ensures that all elements remain readable and usable regardless of the device. Consider touch-based interfaces for tablets and mobile devices, ensuring that buttons and interactive elements are appropriately sized for touch.

5. Ignoring User Feedback

Mistake: Designing screens without involving end users in the process can lead to interfaces that don't align with the real-world needs of healthcare professionals. Users may encounter issues that designers didn't foresee, and the system may be less effective because it doesn't accommodate the specific workflow or preferences of the users.

Solution: Involve healthcare professionals in the design process from the start. Use user feedback to inform the development and design decisions at each stage. Conduct user testing, including usability studies and focus groups, to identify pain points and areas of improvement. Continuously gather feedback to iterate on the design and refine it based on real-world usage.

6. Poor Data Visualization

Mistake: In healthcare, data visualization is key to presenting complex information in a way that's clear and easy to understand. Using overly complicated charts or displaying too much data at once can confuse users and lead to mistakes. For example, displaying patient vitals or test results in a text-heavy format without clear graphical representation can make it harder for healthcare professionals to spot trends or anomalies.

Solution: Use clear, intuitive data visualizations such as charts, graphs, and colour-coded indicators to present key information. Ensure that each visualization is easy to interpret at a glance and avoids information overload. Implement clear labels, legends, and tooltips that help users understand the data at a glance. Consider the context in which the data will be used—healthcare professionals often need to identify trends or anomalies quickly, so the visuals should highlight the most important information.

7. Lack of Error Prevention and Feedback

Mistake: Failing to provide proper error prevention mechanisms or feedback when something goes wrong is a common mistake in UI design. Healthcare professionals need to be immediately alerted when an error occurs—whether it's inputting incorrect data or a system malfunction—and should be given clear guidance on how to resolve the issue.

Solution: Implement real-time error detection and validation for data input fields, providing immediate feedback to users. For example, if a nurse enters a patient's birthdate incorrectly, the system should highlight the error and suggest corrections. Use visual cues such as colour changes (e.g., red highlights) or pop-up messages to ensure that users are aware of errors. Additionally, provide clear instructions or guidance on how to fix mistakes without frustrating the user.

8. Overcomplicated Forms

Mistake: Forms that require extensive data entry, such as patient intake forms or medication orders, can be a source of frustration if they are too lengthy or complicated. Healthcare professionals may have to fill out long, tedious forms while multitasking, and any unnecessary fields or steps increase the risk of errors.

Solution: Simplify forms by removing unnecessary fields and breaking long forms into smaller, manageable sections. Use conditional logic to show or hide fields based on previous answers, minimising the number of options users need to interact with.

Where possible, automate data entry through auto fill or integration with other systems to speed up the process and reduce errors.

9. Inadequate Accessibility

Mistake: Failing to design HIS interfaces with accessibility in mind can exclude healthcare professionals with disabilities or impair their ability to use the system efficiently. For example, relying solely on colour to convey information can be problematic for users with colour blindness.

Solution: Follow accessibility guidelines such as the Web Content Accessibility Guidelines (WCAG) to ensure your design accommodates users with disabilities. Provide options for screen readers, keyboard navigation, and colour contrast adjustments. Ensure that font sizes are adjustable, and avoid relying on colour alone to communicate important information. By designing with accessibility in mind, you can ensure that all users have an equal opportunity to interact with the HIS effectively.

Conclusion

Effective UI design in Health Information Systems is not just about aesthetics, it directly influences usability, workflow efficiency, and patient safety. By avoiding common pitfalls such as clutter, poor navigation, and lack of accessibility, designers can create systems that empower healthcare professionals rather than hinder them. Ultimately, thoughtful and user-centred design leads to safer, more reliable, and more efficient healthcare delivery.

References:

1. Nielsen, J. (1994). *Usability engineering.* Morgan Kaufmann.
2. Shneiderman, B., Plaisant, C., Cohen, M., Jacobs, S., Elmqvist, N., & Diakopoulos, N. (2016). *Designing the user interface: Strategies for effective human-computer interaction* (6th ed.). Pearson.

Chapter 02: Guidelines for UX Design in Health Information Systems: Principles, Practices, and Pitfalls

When designing Health Information Systems (HIS), the key to success lies in creating interfaces that are user-friendly, efficient, and truly aligned with the needs of healthcare professionals. A user interface (UI) is not just a tool to input data but a bridge between clinicians and technology, enabling better patient care and streamlined workflows. In this chapter, we'll discuss two fundamental guidelines for designing effective screens for HIS: **Involving the User** and **Anticipating the User's Needs**. These principles will serve as the foundation for creating systems that are intuitive, practical, and enhance the overall experience for healthcare professionals.

1. Involve the User

Mistake: Designing interfaces without fully understanding the end users' requirements is a common pitfall. Healthcare professionals are the primary users of HIS, and their input is essential throughout the design process to ensure the system meets their needs.

Solution: The first and most crucial step in designing any HIS screen is understanding the user's workflow, tasks, and constraints. Involving users at every stage of the design process ensures that the screens are intuitive and efficient. A user-centred design approach means that feedback from actual users—clinicians, nurses, administrators, and other healthcare staff—must be incorporated at multiple stages.

Key Stages for Involving Users:

- **Early Design Phase**: Begin by brainstorming with users to understand their requirements. Create initial mock-ups and gather user feedback to iterate on the design.
- **Prototyping Phase**: Allow users to test the interface at this stage. By interacting with the prototype, they can provide feedback on usability, functionality, and overall user experience.
- **Before Delivery**: Conduct functional testing to identify any issues with the screens before the final product is delivered. This phase ensures that the design works as intended and meets user expectations.
- **Post-Implementation**: Once the system is live, gather feedback from users to identify any challenges they face.

Use this information to refine the design for future updates and releases.

Understanding the Diversity of Users:

An HIS is not used by just one type of professional. There are multiple users involved in the system, each with their own needs and responsibilities. For example, clinicians, nurses, receptionists, pharmacists, and administrators all interact with the system differently. By understanding these different user roles and workflows, designers can create screens that cater to the specific needs of each role. Regular design review meetings should include use-case scenarios to ensure that the system aligns with the clinical workflows and practices followed by the institution.

Use Case Scenario:

Consider a small clinic that requires software for registration, prescribing, and dispensing medications. While this may seem like a straightforward project, it involves multiple roles—receptionists, clinicians, pharmacists, and inventory managers—each of whom interacts with the system in different ways. During the requirements phase, the design team should work closely with the clinic's team to document the specific needs of each user and understand the clinic's workflow. By discussing these use cases and incorporating feedback from all users, the design team can create a system that's efficient and user-friendly for everyone involved.

2. Anticipate the User's Needs

Mistake: A common mistake is assuming that users will instinctively know where to find the information they need or how to use a feature. HIS screens must anticipate the needs of healthcare professionals by providing relevant information upfront, without requiring users to search or guess.

Solution: Anticipation is especially important in healthcare settings where time is often critical, and mistakes can have serious consequences. The interface should be designed so that users can quickly access the information they need without unnecessary clicks or confusion. Providing links to relevant medical knowledge, patient data, or clinical guidelines directly on the screen helps users make informed decisions more quickly, minimising errors.

Key Considerations for Anticipating User Needs:

- **Concise Information**: The system should display only the most relevant data for the task at hand, reducing information overload and enabling users to focus on what matters most.

- **Quick Access to Critical Information**: Healthcare professionals often need to make time-sensitive decisions. Ensure that key information, such as patient medical history or allergy alerts, is immediately accessible without the need to search through multiple screens.
- **Clear Visual Cues**: Use icons, tooltips, and visual cues to guide users. For example, hover-over text should explain the purpose of icons, so users understand their function and are more likely to interact with them.

Use Case Scenario:

Consider a **Medication Administration** module where a nurse is about to administer intravenous fluids to a patient. Before proceeding, the nurse needs to verify the patient's medical history and check for any allergies. To streamline this process, the system includes an icon next to the patient's ID that, when clicked, displays the patient's drug profile.

However, if the icon does not clearly communicate its purpose (e.g., by showing a tooltip such as 'Patient Drug Profile' when hovered over), the nurse might overlook it, assuming it is just a generic symbol. This could delay critical decision-making. A simple improvement—ensuring the icon provides a clear description upon hover—can make the system more intuitive, reducing the chance of errors and improving overall efficiency. This is just one example of how anticipating users' needs and making their tasks easier can improve system usability.

When designing Health Information Systems (HIS), creating intuitive, efficient, and error-free interfaces is essential for improving the quality of healthcare delivery. This chapter focuses on three important design principles: **Anticipating the User's Needs**, **Maintaining Consistency**, and **Designing Explorable Interfaces**. By adhering to these principles, we ensure that HIS screens help users navigate their tasks swiftly and with confidence, ultimately improving patient care and operational efficiency.

3. Anticipate the User's Needs

Mistake: Failing to inform the user about ongoing processes, such as a search or data retrieval, can lead to confusion and frustration. For example, if a user is searching for a specific patient record from a database of 6,000 records, they may not know if the search process is actively being performed unless there is a clear indication from the system.

Solution: To avoid user confusion, the interface should provide status updates during tasks such as searches or data retrieval. Using visual indicators—such as an icon displaying 'Search in Process... Please wait'—can keep users informed about what is happening in the background. This allows the user to feel in control and aware of the system's progress. Without such feedback, users might prematurely cancel the search and revert to manual methods, assuming that the system is not working.

Key Considerations for Anticipating User Needs:

- **Status Mechanisms**: Displaying indicators, progress bars, or loading animations ensures that users know when a task is in progress, reducing uncertainty.
- **Help Options**: Provide users with easily accessible help options. For instance, an online help button or tooltips can guide users when they are unsure about specific tasks, such as how to execute a process like inventory procurement.

Use Case Scenario:

Consider a **Pharmacy Outpatient Dispensing Module**. A pharmacist is dispensing medication but discovers that the required medication is not available on the tray and must be fetched from inventory. If the pharmacist is unsure how to quickly access the inventory system, this could delay the process, leading to longer waiting times for patients and potential negative impacts on hospital metrics. By including simple online help instructions in the system, such as step-by-step guidance for quickly locating inventory, the pharmacist can proceed efficiently, reducing patient wait times and improving workflow.

4. Maintain Consistency in Design

Mistake: Inconsistent layouts, terminologies, and workflows across different modules can confuse users, especially when they are working under time pressure. For example, if a clinician accesses both the clinical and medication administration modules, they might face difficulty if the screen layout for placing orders is different between the two modules.

Solution: Consistency is key when designing HIS interfaces. A uniform layout, consistent labelling, and similar navigation structures across the system will help reduce cognitive load and confusion. When users interact with the system, they should not have to relearn the interface every time they switch between modules or functions.

Key Considerations for Maintaining Consistency:

- **Consistent Layouts**: Ensure that the placement of buttons, menus, and other UI elements is consistent across all modules.
- **Uniform Terminology**: Use the same terminology throughout the system, particularly when referring to medical terms or data fields, to avoid misunderstandings.
- **Consistent Navigation**: The placement of navigation elements, such as menu bars or links, should be uniform across the system to help users easily orient themselves.

Use Case Scenario:

In a **Clinical and Medication Administration Module**, a clinician might need to place an order for a medication while reviewing patient data. If the screen layout for placing orders in the Medication Administration Module is complex and significantly different from the clinician's usual ordering interface, this may cause confusion. A clinician who is accustomed to the simpler ordering process in the Clinical Module might struggle to adapt to the more complex Medication Administration interface, leading to delays in patient treatment.

To avoid this, ensuring a consistent design across both modules—using the same layout, terminology, and navigation patterns—would help the clinician perform their tasks more efficiently. Consistent design also reduces the likelihood of user frustration and delays.

5. Design Explorable Interfaces to Increase User Efficiency

Mistake: Overloading users with options and information without providing the ability to explore or tailor the interface to their needs can lead to confusion and decreased productivity.

Solution: Design interfaces that allow for Customisation and exploration without overwhelming users. Giving users control over what they see and how they interact with the system can significantly increase their productivity. However, the Customisation should be guided and should not interfere with the overall workflow. Providing clear options for Customisation—such as favourite lists, personalized treatment protocols, and medical knowledge links—can empower users to tailor the interface to suit their specific needs, improving decision-making and efficiency.

Key Considerations for Designing Explorable Interfaces:

- **Customisation**: Allow users to personalize the interface according to their needs, but avoid overwhelming them with excessive Customisation options.

- **Reversible Actions**: Ensure that users can undo or reverse actions when experimenting with the interface. This reduces the fear of making errors and allows users to explore the system without hesitation.

- **User Control**: The system should respond to user actions in a predictable way, and users should feel that they are in control of the task environment.

Use Case Scenario:

A **clinician** frequently accesses the **Clinical Module** for recording patient medical histories and making treatment decisions. By allowing the clinician to customize their homepage—such as by adding patient lists, medical history summaries, or relevant medical links—the clinician can streamline their workflow and make decisions faster. However, the clinician should only be allowed to customize their own interface. Allowing Customisation in shared modules, like the Pharmacy Module, could disrupt communication between users and lead to confusion.

Additionally, **explorable interfaces** are vital for enhancing work efficiency. For example, providing **undo** options for accidental actions (such as mistakenly deleting a medication order) can ensure that users do not become hesitant to explore new features. This functionality supports both novice and expert users by minimising the risk of errors and enhancing overall productivity.

6. Create Designs Which Help Users Minimize, Identify, and Rectify Errors

The primary goal in designing Health Information Systems is to prevent user errors. Errors in health information systems, such as entering duplicate patient details, scheduling overlapping appointments, or booking the same bed for multiple patients, can have serious consequences, including clinical risk. Therefore, the design must be intuitive and help prevent these types of errors through clear, informative error messages. Additionally, error recovery mechanisms should be in place to help users' correct mistakes easily and continue their work.

Consider the following scenario:

a. Imagine a situation where a user accidentally books overlapping appointments for two different patients: *Patient A* from 10:00 to 10:15 AM, and *Patient B* from 10:10 to 10:20 AM. The system should immediately display an error message saying, "You cannot schedule overlapping appointments," with an 'OK' action button. Upon clicking 'OK,' the system should display available time slots again, allowing the user to select a different time for the appointments. This approach ensures that the user can quickly correct the mistake and continue their work without feeling frustrated.

b. Another example could be booking beds for patients. When a user books a bed for a patient (e.g., Bed No. 5 for *Patient A*), the system should automatically disable that bed slot, making it unavailable for other bookings. This proactive design minimizes the chance of double-booking, reducing errors and improving efficiency.

Furthermore, using highlights to indicate errors can be an effective way to guide the user. For instance, if a mandatory field is missing or a wrong entry is made, the system should highlight the error. Once the error is corrected, the highlight should be removed, signalling to the user that the issue has been resolved.

7. Protect the User's Work and Provide a Provision to Track the Status of Work

A crucial aspect of health information system design is ensuring the protection of user work and data privacy. Unauthorized access must be prevented, and the system should adhere to data protection laws, including the Data Protection Act (DPA). This is especially critical for health data, as patient confidentiality is a top priority. Ensuring that only authorized users can access sensitive data through the use of unique passwords or codes is essential to maintaining security.

Consider the following use case scenario for good design:

a. Imagine a doctor who logs in at 9:00 AM to consult with a patient and then accesses an external medical link for additional information. Before the doctor can complete the session, an urgent call requires them to leave. The doctor logs off at 9:30 AM, and the system logs the session's end. Later, when the doctor logs back in at 11:30 AM, the system remembers where the doctor left off—displaying the same medical link that was being referred to earlier. This feature ensures that users don't lose progress and can continue their work from where they last stopped, improving efficiency and user satisfaction.

In addition, tracking the state of the user's work is vital. For example, the system should record when users log in and out, and what actions they have performed. This provides an overview of the user's session, which is especially helpful for clinicians who may need to pick up where they left off, ensuring that there is no loss of critical information or work progress.

8. Provide Visible Navigation

Navigating patient data effectively is one of the most significant challenges in health information system design. With the vast amount of clinical information, it is essential to simplify navigation so that users can access the necessary data quickly and efficiently. A common solution to this issue is to provide a navigational hierarchy on every page, such as a breadcrumb trail. This enables users to track their location within the system and return to the previous page without unnecessary clicks.

Consider the following example for web-based navigation:

Imagine a patient using a health information system to manage appointments. The system includes several pages:

- Manage appointments
- Book appointments

- Reschedule appointments
- Cancel appointments
- Check medical history

If the patient is on the *Cancel appointments* page and wants to book a new appointment, the breadcrumb trail would show the path:

Manage appointments >> Book >> Reschedule >> Cancel

By simply clicking the *Book* hyperlink in the breadcrumb trail, the patient can quickly return to the *Book appointments* page and make a new appointment. Without this navigation tool, the patient would have to use the 'Back' button repeatedly, leading to a cumbersome user experience.

Additionally, providing an overview of the system through a sitemap can be useful for users who might get lost. While sitemaps are not frequently used by all users, they can be helpful in times when users are unsure of their location within the system. Jakob Nielsen's Sitemap usability research indicates that sitemaps offer a quick and simple way to navigate large systems, improving the overall user experience.

9. Train the End User

Training is a crucial step in the successful adoption of Health Information Systems (HIS). Although end-users may be involved in the design process, it is essential to provide training once the system is implemented. Training ensures that users, especially healthcare professionals who may not be tech-savvy, understand how to use the system effectively. Practical hands-on experience with the system's features is necessary for efficient task completion and for realising the benefits of the system.

For hospital information systems, the user demographic may include elderly individuals and experienced healthcare professionals who are not familiar with technology. Therefore, a comprehensive training program is necessary to help these users become comfortable with the system's functionalities. Additionally, providing easy-to-search help documentation and user guides will further support the adoption of the system. Training can significantly reduce confusion, improve usability, and encourage widespread adoption of healthcare IT systems

In conclusion, by focusing on usability, consistency, and thoughtful design, Health Information Systems can improve efficiency, reduce errors, and provide a better user experience for healthcare professionals, ultimately enhancing patient care.

Do's and Don'ts of UX Design for HIS
How do we credit ourselves as better designers of a HI System? Well, designing usable HIS that leads to achieving meaningful use and in turn, increasing adoption can position us as designers of HIS. So, how should we go about creating good designs? What is that we should follow (do) and what must we abstain from (don'ts) while designing usable Health Management Systems?

Without taking a deep dive into the design ecosystem, let's have an informative look at few important do's and don'ts of UX design for HIS

<u>Do's</u>

1. Keep users informed with status mechanisms

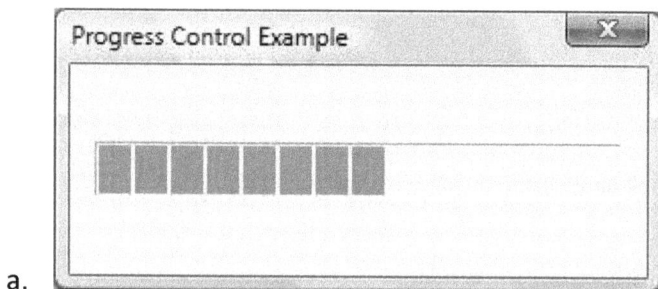

   a.

All Well Management system

Patient Name	Registration.no.	Status of pharmacy order	
Ms. Reece Smith	AR0098079	Completed	✓
Mr. Alistar Rodrigues	AR900567	Completed	✓
Dr. Alen Jones	AR 876435	Completed	✓
Ms. Sandra Bullock	AR23456009	Completed	✓
Mr. George Mattai	AR12345679	Cancelled	
Total Progress			100%

b.

2. Acknowledge the clicking of buttons and reduce the user's wait time

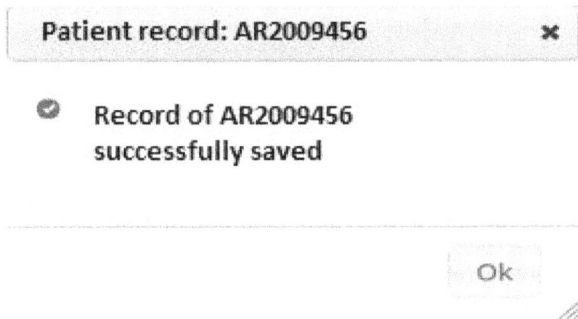

Patient record: AR2009456 ✖

⊘ Record of AR2009456
successfully saved

Ok

a.

3. Provide informative error messages

a.

4. Provide the facility for mouse-over on icons or descriptions

a.

5. Minimize learning curve

6. Provide online help and other resources to tackle issues

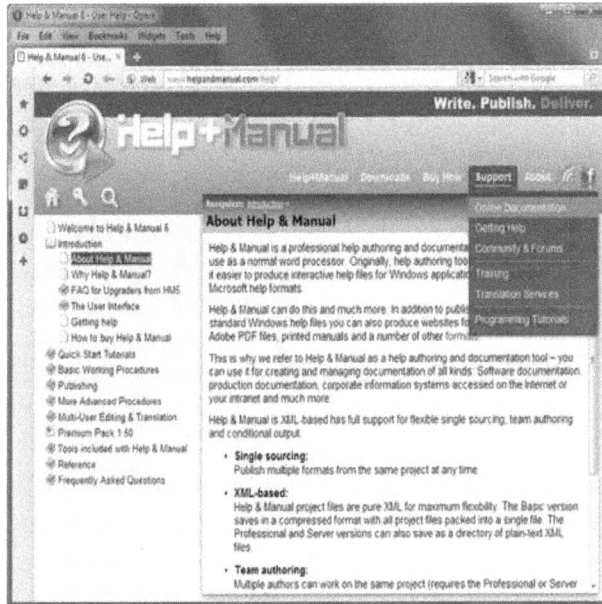

a.

7. Keep display of clinical information as simple as possible

8. Provide a task friendly environment to the user

9. Use relevant medical terminologies wherever applicable

10. Compensate colour blindness by using secondary cues

11. Ensure design supports readability

12. Bring to the user all the information and tools required to perform the task

13. Maintain consistency in design

14. Use responsive and intelligent defaults.

15. Keep the users occupied thereby increasing their efficiency at work

16. Allow reversible actions

34

17. Protect users' work

18. Provide visible navigation.

Don'ts

1. Do not let the user's actions occur without any system response.

2. Do not allow the user to guess the time left to complete the action

3. Do not make the user search for relevant task information

4. Do not make the design complicated for novice users

5. Do not provide irrelevant and unnecessary information

6. Do not use unnecessary graphics

7. Do not use too many technical jargon, be it information or error messages

8. Do not use same menus, icons and buttons to represent different actions

9. Do not use small fonts

10. Do not choose icons that are hard to interpret

11. Do not use abbreviations in the design unless necessary

12. Do not place commands or icons too closely together, as they may cancel each other. For example, placing the delete and OK buttons very side by side can lead to accidental deletion of the action

13. Do not use invisible navigational structures

14. Do not create a help system that is difficult to navigate

15. Do not design a system that cannot save or recover.

16. Do not make the design so difficult that the recovered files are hard to locate.

17. Do not design such that users have to re-enter the same data several times

18. Do not use ambiguous messages to indicate errors

19. Do not allow the user to make multiple errors without notification

20. Do not allow the user to proceed further without acknowledging the error.

These will be elaborated in Chapter 4.

References:

1. Kushniruk, A. W., & Patel, V. L. (2004). Cognitive and usability engineering methods for the evaluation of clinical information systems *Journal of Biomedical Informatics, 37*(1), 56–76. https://doi.org/10.1016/j.jbi.2004.01.003
2. Jones, P. H. (2013). *Design for care: Innovating healthcare experience*. Rosenfeld Media.
3. Gray, K., & Lederman, R. (Eds.). (2025). *Research handbook on health information systems: Theories and methods.* Edward Elgar Publishing.

Chapter 03: Guidelines for GUI Design in Health Information Systems: Usability, Workflow, and Patient Safety

Designing effective graphical user interfaces (GUIs) for Health Information Systems (HIS) extends far beyond mere aesthetic considerations. It constitutes a critical component in enhancing usability, promoting patient safety, and ensuring operational efficiency within healthcare environments. In high-stakes clinical settings, where timely access to accurate information is paramount, the design of the interface through which users interact with the system can significantly influence both workflow effectiveness and clinical decision-making.

A thoughtfully constructed GUI not only facilitates intuitive navigation and data entry but also reduces cognitive load, thereby alleviating clinician fatigue and lowering the risk of user-induced errors. These benefits directly contribute to improved patient outcomes, particularly in contexts where rapid interpretation and response are required. Moreover, usability issues in HIS have been linked to workarounds, decreased user satisfaction, and even adverse events, further underscoring the necessity for rigorous attention to interface design.

This chapter delineates a set of usability-centred guidelines tailored specifically to the design of GUIs in the context of HIS. These guidelines are firmly rooted in human-centred design principles, which prioritise the needs, limitations, and behaviours of end users throughout the development process. Furthermore, they account for the distinctive characteristics and constraints of healthcare workflows, including interdisciplinary collaboration, time-sensitive decision-making, and the need for interoperability across diverse clinical systems By integrating these principles, designers can create interfaces that not only support but actively enhance the quality and safety of healthcare delivery.

1. User-Centred Design (UCD) is Foundational

At the core of effective graphical user interface (GUI) development for Health Information Systems (HIS) lies the principle of User-Centred Design (UCD). This methodological approach prioritises the needs, behaviours, and limitations of the end-users throughout the entire design and development lifecycle. In the context of healthcare, these users encompass a diverse range of stakeholders, including clinicians (e.g., physicians, nurses, allied health professionals), administrative personnel, and, in certain contexts, patients themselves. As such, designing interfaces that truly serve their intended purpose requires a deep and nuanced understanding of the distinct tasks, pressures, and cognitive demands faced by these individuals.

Usability cannot be achieved in abstraction; it begins with a comprehensive exploration of the clinical environment in which the HIS will be deployed. This necessitates the implementation of **contextual inquiry**, a qualitative research method involving direct observation of users within their natural work settings. By witnessing real-time interactions with current systems and workflows, designers can uncover latent needs, recurrent challenges, and contextual nuances that may not be captured through interviews or surveys alone.

Equally critical is the **early and sustained engagement of stakeholders**. Involving end-users—particularly clinicians—during the initial stages of design and throughout iterative testing phases fosters a sense of ownership and ensures the interface aligns with practical realities. This participatory approach helps to surface implicit knowledge and tacit expectations that may otherwise be overlooked, and it enables the early identification of design flaws or mismatches between system behaviour and user intent.

Furthermore, the development process must be informed by well-defined **user personas** and **task models**. These representations of archetypal users, such as nurses, general practitioners, emergency physicians, or laboratory technicians, serve as focal points for design decisions. By mapping interface elements to actual user roles and associated tasks, designers can create GUIs that support efficiency, reduce cognitive friction, and cater to domain-specific requirements. This task-oriented design philosophy is particularly important in healthcare settings, where responsibilities, workflows, and information needs can vary significantly across roles.

Ultimately, the adoption of UCD principles in HIS interface design not only enhances usability but also promotes system adoption, reduces training overhead, and supports safer and more effective patient care.

2. Support Cognitive Workflows, Not Just Data Entry

Health Information Systems (HIS) must be designed with a recognition that clinical work extends far beyond the act of data entry. Clinicians are engaged in complex cognitive activities, including the interpretation of diverse information sources, the synthesis of clinical data, and the formulation of time-sensitive decisions that directly impact patient outcomes. Therefore, graphical user interfaces (GUIs) must be purposefully designed to support these cognitive workflows, rather than simply serving as repositories for data input.

Traditional information systems often prioritise data capture and storage, neglecting the nuanced ways in which users think, reason, and interact with clinical content. This disconnect can result in interfaces that hinder rather than help clinical decision-making. A cognitive-centric approach to GUI design acknowledges that clinicians need to see patterns, detect anomalies, and draw connections quickly and accurately—activities that require more than just structured fields and drop-down menus.

To this end, **task-based layouts** should be employed, wherein screens are organised according to specific clinical functions or workflows—such as order entry, patient review, diagnostic reasoning, or discharge planning—rather than by system modules or database structures. This alignment enables users to remain task-focused, reducing the need for unnecessary navigation and mental switching between disparate interface components.

Additionally, GUIs should be optimised to **facilitate rapid visual scanning**, allowing users to extract essential information at a glance. This can be achieved through the strategic use of visual design principles, including **grouping related elements**,

incorporating appropriate whitespace, and establishing **clear visual hierarchies**. Such design features help users to prioritise relevant information and avoid missing critical cues, particularly in high-pressure clinical environments where time is constrained and interruptions are frequent.

A fundamental principle in this context is the **minimisation of cognitive load**. Interfaces that present excessive amounts of information simultaneously can overwhelm users, impairing their ability to process and act upon what is presented. Progressive disclosure, intelligent filtering, and context-sensitive displays can be employed to present the right information at the right time, thereby supporting mental clarity and reducing the risk of error.

In sum, GUI design in HIS must be grounded in a deep understanding of clinical cognition. By aligning interface structures with the mental models and workflows of healthcare professionals, designers can create systems that enhance clinical reasoning, improve efficiency, and ultimately contribute to safer and more effective care delivery.

3. Ensure Information is Accessible and Actionable

In the design of graphical user interfaces (GUIs) for Health Information Systems (HIS), the accessibility and actionability of information are of paramount importance. Clinical environments are often characterised by high cognitive demand, time pressure, and the necessity for rapid, informed decision-making. As such, interfaces must be designed to ensure that critical patient information is not only readily available but also easily interpretable and immediately actionable.

The capacity to swiftly locate and comprehend pertinent data—such as vital signs, laboratory results, medication orders, or clinical alerts—can directly influence patient safety and care quality. Information overload, poorly organised displays, or ambiguous visual cues can significantly impede clinical reasoning and increase the risk of errors. To mitigate these risks, systems must be designed to **highlight critical or abnormal values** in a manner that draws appropriate attention without contributing to visual fatigue or alarm desensitisation. For instance, **colour-coding** may be employed to flag abnormalities—such as red for critical deviations—however, this must be implemented judiciously. Overuse of colour can dilute its effectiveness and compromise accessibility for users with colour vision deficiencies. Thus, colour should be supplemented by additional visual or textual indicators where possible.

Another key consideration is the capacity for **customisable views**. Given the diversity of roles within clinical teams—and the corresponding variability in information needs—interfaces should support user-specific tailoring. Allowing users to configure dashboards or data panels according to their workflow enables them to focus on the information most relevant to their clinical tasks. For example, a nurse may prioritise real-time monitoring data, while a physician may require longitudinal trends or diagnostic summaries. Personalisation enhances efficiency, reduces information clutter, and promotes a sense of control and engagement with the system.

Furthermore, effective GUIs should support **drill-down navigation**, whereby users are initially presented with high-level summaries but can easily access more granular details as required. This layered approach to information presentation respects the cognitive principles of progressive disclosure, allowing users to engage with complex data at a manageable pace. For example, a dashboard may present an overview of a patient's condition with key indicators, each of which can be expanded to reveal underlying data, such as historical lab trends or narrative clinical notes. This not only supports informed decision-making but also improves transparency and traceability within the clinical record.

In summary, ensuring that information is both accessible and actionable requires a careful balance between visibility, clarity, and user control. Interfaces that foreground critical information, offer user-driven customisation, and facilitate intuitive navigation through layers of data are better positioned to support timely and accurate clinical judgement in demanding healthcare contexts.

4. Design for Safety and Error Prevention

In the context of healthcare, usability transcends convenience and becomes a matter of patient safety. Poorly designed graphical user interfaces (GUIs) can contribute directly to clinical errors, which may compromise patient outcomes. As such, the design of healthcare interfaces must prioritise safety and integrate mechanisms to minimise the potential for user error.

A critical design strategy involves the judicious use of confirmation dialogues, particularly for high-risk actions such as prescribing or discontinuing medications. While overuse of confirmations can lead to alert fatigue, their selective application in contexts with serious clinical implications can act as a valuable safeguard against inadvertent actions.

Preventing wrong-patient errors is another essential consideration. Interfaces should prominently display key patient identifiers, including full name, photograph (where available), and a unique patient ID, throughout the user journey. This persistent visibility supports accurate patient identification and reduces the likelihood of clinicians performing actions on the incorrect record.

Moreover, systems should support error recovery through features such as undo functionality and reversible actions where feasible. Allowing users to easily correct mistakes without requiring administrative intervention not only reduces cognitive load but also enhances trust in the system and encourages safe usage behaviours.

Ultimately, designing for safety and error prevention necessitates a comprehensive understanding of clinical workflows, human factors, and the cognitive demands placed on healthcare professionals. By embedding safety-oriented design principles within GUIs, developers can contribute meaningfully to the reduction of avoidable harm in healthcare settings.

5. Follow Consistency and Standards

Consistency is a cornerstone of effective interface design, particularly within the high-stakes environment of Health Information Systems (HIS). When users encounter predictable and uniform patterns across a system, cognitive effort is reduced, recognition is enhanced, and the potential for error is minimised. Consistent design facilitates more efficient learning, improves user satisfaction, and fosters trust in the system's reliability—critical factors in healthcare settings where rapid and accurate information processing is vital.

One of the most effective ways to achieve consistency is through the adoption of **familiar user interface (UI) patterns**. These patterns—whether derived from platform-specific guidelines (e.g., web-based UI toolkits or operating system conventions) or industry standards—serve as cognitive shortcuts, enabling users to intuitively navigate and interact with the interface. In the context of healthcare, alignment with established norms such as those informed by **HL7 (Health Level Seven International)** and **FHIR (Fast Healthcare Interoperability Resources)** is especially important. These frameworks not only support consistency in interface behaviour but also ensure interoperability and semantic coherence across different systems and institutions.

Another critical element of consistent design is the use of **standardised medical terminology**. The language employed within HIS must be clinically accurate, unambiguous, and appropriate to the user's level of expertise. Consistency in terminology—such as using "myocardial infarction" rather than alternating with "heart attack"—helps avoid confusion and supports precise clinical documentation and communication. Integration with controlled vocabularies and coding systems such as **SNOMED CT** or **ICD-10** further enhances data quality and facilitates secondary uses of clinical data, including research and audit.

In addition, **standardisation of layout elements** is essential to ensure a coherent and intuitive user experience. Buttons, icons, menus, and other interactive elements should maintain consistent positioning, appearance, and functionality across all screens within the system. For instance, commonly used actions—such as "save," "cancel," or "submit"—should be located in predictable positions and follow uniform labelling and iconography. This reduces the need for users to relearn interface components on different pages or modules, thereby improving task efficiency and reducing the likelihood of unintended actions.

In sum, adherence to consistency and standards in GUI design not only simplifies user interaction but also contributes to system safety, usability, and interoperability. By leveraging established UI conventions, standardised clinical language, and uniform interface elements, designers can create more predictable, trustworthy, and user-friendly Health Information Systems that support the complex cognitive and collaborative demands of healthcare environments.

6. Design for Time-Critical Tasks

Healthcare environments are often characterised by high intensity and time-sensitive decision-making. Clinicians frequently operate under significant time pressures, particularly in acute and emergency care settings. In such contexts, the efficiency of graphical user interfaces (GUIs) is paramount. Interfaces must be optimised to facilitate rapid, intuitive interaction in order to support clinical workflows without introducing delays or cognitive burdens that could compromise patient care.

A fundamental principle in designing for time-critical tasks is the reduction of unnecessary user actions. Interfaces should be engineered to minimise the number of clicks, keystrokes, and navigation steps required to complete routine processes, such as charting, medication prescribing, or discharge planning. Streamlining these high-frequency tasks not only saves valuable time but also reduces the likelihood of user fatigue and associated errors.

The incorporation of keyboard shortcuts is another effective strategy to enhance efficiency, particularly in high-throughput settings such as emergency departments or intensive care units. When implemented appropriately, keyboard commands can expedite task execution and offer an alternative to mouse-based navigation, which may be slower or impractical in fast-paced clinical environments.

Furthermore, the use of pre-populated data, where clinically appropriate and safe, can significantly reduce input time. Leveraging defaults based on clinical guidelines or auto-filling fields with information from previous encounters can expedite documentation and decision-making processes. However, such features must be implemented with caution, ensuring that clinicians retain the ability to verify and modify pre-filled information to maintain accuracy and avoid propagation of errors.

In summary, GUIs designed for time-critical healthcare tasks must prioritise speed, clarity, and user control. By reducing interaction overhead and supporting clinician efficiency, these interfaces can play a crucial role in facilitating timely and effective patient care.

7. Accommodate a Variety of User Expertise

Health Information Systems (HIS) are utilised by a diverse range of users with varying degrees of clinical experience, digital literacy, and familiarity with specific technologies. This heterogeneity presents a significant challenge for interface design, necessitating flexible solutions that accommodate both novice and expert users without compromising usability or functionality. A one-size-fits-all approach is unlikely to meet the needs of such a varied user base; instead, GUI design must be adaptable, supportive, and inclusive.

One of the most effective strategies for addressing differences in user expertise is the implementation of **progressive disclosure**. This design principle involves initially presenting users with only the most essential and frequently used information or functionality, while offering more advanced options or detailed data upon request. By doing so, cognitive overload is minimised for less experienced users, who are not burdened with complex features they may not yet need or understand, while experienced users retain access to deeper system capabilities. For example, a basic patient summary may be displayed by default, with expandable panels offering access to full clinical histories, diagnostic reports, or decision support tools as needed.

In parallel, it is essential to incorporate **on boarding mechanisms and contextual help tools** that facilitate user learning and promote system adoption. Features such as inline guidance, interactive tooltips, walk-through tutorials, and embedded training modules can assist users in navigating unfamiliar workflows and discovering system functionalities. These tools are particularly beneficial during initial exposure to the system or following major updates. Moreover, the inclusion of context-sensitive support reduces reliance on external documentation or training sessions, allowing users to resolve issues or learn new tasks within the interface itself.

Another key consideration is the need to **adapt interfaces to different devices and user roles**. Modern healthcare environments increasingly rely on a variety of platforms, including desktop workstations, tablets, and mobile devices, each of which may be preferred depending on the clinical context or user role. For instance, ward nurses may require quick access to patient charts via tablets during rounds, while consultants may perform in-depth reviews on desktop systems Accordingly, interfaces must be **responsive and role-aware**, ensuring that layout, functionality, and performance remain optimal across device types and are aligned with the specific needs of the user. This includes scalable designs, adaptive content prioritisation, and input methods suited to the device in use.

Ultimately, accommodating a broad spectrum of user expertise enhances not only usability but also equity in technology access. By designing for variability, systems can support confident and effective use across the entire spectrum of healthcare professionals, thereby improving clinical efficiency, reducing training burdens, and fostering a more inclusive digital environment in healthcare delivery.

8. Incorporate Feedback and Iteration

Usability within healthcare systems is not a static attribute but rather an evolving quality that must be continually assessed and improved. The dynamic nature of clinical environments, coupled with the diversity of user needs and workflows, necessitates an iterative approach to interface design. Ongoing refinement informed by real-world use is essential to ensure that graphical user interfaces (GUIs) remain effective, intuitive, and aligned with clinical practice.

Regular usability testing is a cornerstone of this iterative process. Employing methodologies such as think-aloud protocols, heuristic evaluations, and high-fidelity simulations can yield valuable insights into how users interact with the system. These methods allow designers to identify usability issues that may not be apparent during initial development phases and to observe how clinicians navigate complex tasks under realistic conditions.

In addition to structured testing, it is vital to establish mechanisms for capturing user feedback directly within the system. Enabling clinicians to flag confusing or inefficient interface elements in real time encourages a participatory design culture and ensures that end-users have a voice in the development process. This approach also facilitates the identification of context-specific issues that may only emerge during actual clinical use.

Agile development methodologies are particularly well-suited to supporting rapid iteration and continuous usability enhancement. By promoting short development cycles, frequent stakeholder engagement, and responsiveness to feedback, agile approaches enable more timely and targeted improvements. Such flexibility is especially important in healthcare settings, where evolving clinical demands and regulatory requirements may necessitate regular updates to system functionality and design.

In conclusion, the incorporation of feedback and iterative design is essential to maintaining high usability standards in healthcare interfaces. A sustained commitment to evaluation, user involvement, and responsive development practices ensures that digital tools remain fit for purpose, safe, and conducive to high-quality patient care.

9. Support Interoperability and Integration

In the increasingly interconnected healthcare landscape, **interoperability** and **system integration** are essential for creating a seamless and efficient workflow. Health Information Systems (HIS) are rarely standalone entities; rather, they must interact with a multitude of other systems, ranging from electronic health records (EHRs) to laboratory information systems, radiology systems, pharmacy databases, and more. A key challenge in designing graphical user interfaces (GUIs) is ensuring that data from these diverse sources is presented clearly, coherently, and in a way that supports the clinical decision-making process.

Unifying interfaces is one of the most effective ways to address this challenge. It is crucial to avoid creating what is often referred to as the "swivel-chair" experience—where clinicians must switch between multiple disparate systems to gather relevant information. This not only disrupts workflow but can also lead to delays, errors, and frustration. To mitigate this, GUIs should aim to integrate data from multiple systems into a unified interface, enabling users to view and interact with information without unnecessary navigation between separate platforms This can be achieved through techniques such as **data aggregation**, where disparate data sources are merged into a single, cohesive interface that presents a holistic view of the patient's status and care trajectory.

In addition, **visual consistency across integrated modules** is paramount. Even when pulling data from third-party systems, the integrated interface should maintain uniformity in terms of layout, colour schemes, typography, and iconography. This consistency reduces cognitive load and helps users mentally map the integrated data to familiar visual cues, facilitating quicker understanding and action. For example, if data from a third-party laboratory system is displayed within the HIS, it should use the same colour scheme, font, and button placement as the primary

HIS interface. Such design coherence ensures that users do not have to relearn how to interpret data, regardless of its source, and can more easily assimilate information into their workflow.

Furthermore, **highlighting the source of data** is essential to maintaining transparency and trust in the system. Given that healthcare data often originates from a range of systems with varying levels of reliability and accuracy, it is important to make clear to the user where each piece of information has come from. This could be achieved by incorporating visual indicators, such as labels, icons, or colour-coded tags, that specify the data source (e.g., "Lab result from Hospital A", or "Medication order from EHR system"). This not only helps users assess the validity of the information but also enables them to identify potential discrepancies, such as outdated or incomplete data, and take appropriate action.

Ultimately, ensuring that a GUI supports **interoperability and integration** is crucial for fostering efficient, error-free, and timely decision-making in healthcare settings. By unifying interfaces, maintaining visual consistency, and clearly identifying the source of data, HIS can provide users with a streamlined experience that enhances workflow, reduces the risk of errors, and promotes a more coordinated approach to patient care.

10. Design for Privacy, Security, and Compliance

In healthcare, usability must be balanced with stringent requirements for privacy, data security, and regulatory compliance. Clinical systems handle highly sensitive personal health information, and any compromise in data protection can have serious ethical, legal, and clinical consequences. Therefore, it is imperative that graphical user interfaces (GUIs) not only support efficient and intuitive use but also uphold the highest standards of confidentiality and integrity, in accordance with frameworks such as the General Data Protection Regulation (GDPR) in Europe and the Health Insurance Portability and Accountability Act (HIPAA) in the United States.

Role-based access control (RBAC) is a fundamental mechanism for safeguarding patient information. By tailoring data access according to the specific roles and responsibilities of users—such as physicians, nurses, administrators, or allied health professionals—systems can enforce the principle of least privilege, thereby reducing the risk of unauthorised access. This also enhances usability by limiting on-screen information to what is clinically relevant, thereby reducing cognitive overload and potential error.

Login mechanisms must strike a balance between robust security and user efficiency. Secure yet seamless authentication methods—such as single sign-on (SSO), smart cards, or biometric authentication—can significantly reduce login friction without compromising security. In high-pressure clinical environments, overly complex login procedures may discourage secure practices, leading users to seek workarounds that can undermine system safeguards. Therefore, authentication workflows should be optimised for both security and clinical practicality.

Transparency regarding data access and monitoring is equally vital. Interfaces should clearly communicate the presence and purpose of audit trails—logs that record user actions such as data access, modifications, or deletions. When users are informed that their interactions with patient records are tracked, it reinforces accountability while also building trust in the system's integrity. Moreover, clear communication about data governance can help clinicians understand the rationale behind certain restrictions or system behaviours, thereby improving compliance and acceptance.

In summary, designing for privacy, security, and compliance is a complex but essential component of healthcare interface design. It requires thoughtful integration of regulatory requirements, technical safeguards, and user-centred principles to ensure that systems are both secure and usable in real-world clinical settings.

Conclusion

In conclusion, the design of graphical user interfaces (GUIs) in Health Information Systems (HIS) is inextricably linked to the broader concept of system usability. The effectiveness of a GUI extends far beyond its visual appeal or technological sophistication; it is fundamentally about how well it supports the needs and workflows of its users—healthcare professionals who rely on these systems for decision-making in high-pressure environments. When interface design is suboptimal, the consequences are far-reaching, impacting not only the satisfaction and productivity of users but, more critically, the safety and quality of patient care. Poorly designed interfaces can frustrate users, introduce operational inefficiencies, and increase the likelihood of errors, all of which compromise the ability to deliver timely and accurate care.

Conversely, well-executed GUI design, grounded in the realities of clinical workflows, can greatly enhance both user experience and system performance. By adhering to **human-centred design principles**, developers can create interfaces that are not only visually intuitive but also aligned with the cognitive and operational needs of healthcare practitioners. This approach ensures that the interface supports rather than impedes clinical decision-making, minimises cognitive load, and facilitates efficient access to critical patient data. Such interfaces empower clinicians to make informed, timely decisions, ultimately improving care quality and patient safety.

The integration of these principles—user-centred design, understanding of clinical environments, and attention to usability—enables the development of GUIs that serve as valuable tools within healthcare delivery. When a GUI is intuitive, efficient, and responsive to the needs of diverse healthcare roles, it transforms from a mere data-entry mechanism into a vital component of the clinical workflow. It supports healthcare professionals in their task of providing high-quality, safe, and effective care, thereby contributing to improved patient outcomes.

Ultimately, the development of effective graphical user interfaces for Health Information Systems is not just a design challenge, but a fundamental element in the ongoing advancement of healthcare technology. As HIS continue to evolve, prioritising usability and user-centred design will be key to ensuring that these systems are both functional and supportive, empowering healthcare professionals and improving the overall quality of care.

References:

1. Abramson, E. L., Patel, V., Malhotra, S., Pfoh, E. R., Nena Osorio, S., & Bates, D. W. (2012). Physician experiences transitioning between an older versus newer electronic health record for electronic prescribing. *International Journal of Medical Informatics, 81*(8), 539–548. https://doi.org/10.1016/j.ijmedinf.2012.03.003
2. Ash, J. S., Berg, M., & Coiera, E. (2004). Some unintended consequences of information technology in health care: The nature of patient care information system-related errors. *Journal of the American Medical Informatics Association, 11*(2), 104–112. https://doi.org/10.1197/jamia.M1471
3. Ratwani, R. M., Savage, E., Will, A., Fong, A., Karavite, D., Muthu, N., ... & Hettinger, A. Z. (2018). Identifying electronic health record usability and safety challenges in pediatric settings. *Health Affairs, 37*(11), 1752–1759. https://doi.org/10.1377/hlthaff.2018.0699
4. Zhang, J., Johnson, T. R., Patel, V. L., Paige, D. L., & Kubose, T. (2003). Using usability heuristics to evaluate patient safety of medical devices. *Journal of Biomedical*

Informatics, 36(1–2), 23–30. https://doi.org/10.1016/S1532-0464(03)00060-1

5. Campbell, J. L. (2024). *User experience research and usability of health information technology*. CRC Press.
6. Lippeveld, T., Sauerborn, R., & Bodart, C. (2000). *Design and implementation of health information systeMs* World Health Organization.
7. Lazar, J. (2006). *Web usability: A user-centered design approach*. Addison Wesley.

Chapter 04: Do's and Don'ts of UX Design for Healthcare Information Systems

Designing a Healthcare Information System (HIS) is far more than crafting sleek interfaces or cramming in flashy features. At its heart, it's about building a system that is intuitive, dependable, and genuinely enables healthcare professionals to provide the best possible care. A thoughtfully designed HIS doesn't merely streamline workflows — it lifts the burden on busy clinicians, reduces the risk of errors, enhances communication across teams, and ultimately improves patient outcomes.

When done well, it becomes an indispensable tool that helps doctors, nurses, and staff focus on what truly matters: delivering safe, efficient, and compassionate care — without the added frustration of wrestling with poor design. So, how do we get it right? Here's a straightforward guide to the **do's and don'ts of UX design** for healthcare systems—packed with practical insights, not buzzwords.

Do's

1. **Keep users in the loop**

   Always let users know what's happening, whether it's

loading a patient record or sending a lab request. Progress bars, confirmation messages, or status indicators can go a long way in reducing anxiety.

2. **Give instant, clear feedback**

   When someone clicks a button or submits a form, acknowledge it right away. A simple "Saved successfully" message reassures users that their action worked.

3. **Make error messages helpful**

   Don't leave users guessing. If they've missed a field or entered the wrong data, explain exactly what went wrong and how to fix it.

4. **Use tooltips and labels wisely**

   Provide explanations or hints when people hover over buttons or icons. This is especially helpful for new or occasional users.

5. **Simplify the learning curve**

   Aim for a design that feels intuitive, so users can get started with minimal training.

6. **Offer easy access to help**

   Provide built-in help resources like FAQs, guides, or a searchable Help Centre so users can troubleshoot without calling IT.

7. **Keep clinical content clear and uncluttered**

   Present essential information upfront and avoid overwhelming users with unnecessary details.

8. **Design around real tasks**

   Focus on supporting common workflows so users can get their work done smoothly.

9. **Use accurate medical language**

   When appropriate, stick to standard medical terminology so professionals know exactly what's meant.

10. **Make it colour blind-friendly**

    Don't rely solely on colour to convey information, instead use text labels, shapes, or icons as well.

11. **Prioritise readability**

    Choose legible fonts, appropriate text sizes, and good contrast between text and background.

12. **Group related tools and information together**

    Keep everything needed for a task in one place to avoid constant screen switching.

13. **Keep the design consistent**

    Stick to uniform layouts, colours, and controls throughout the system to help users feel oriented.

14. **Use smart defaults**

    Where possible, pre-fill fields with logical options to save time and reduce errors.

15. **Help users stay focused**

    Design interfaces that keep users engaged, without unnecessary pop-ups or distractions.

16. **Allow undo and cancellation**

    Give users a way to reverse actions to reduce fear of making mistakes.

17. **Protect user work**

    Include auto save functions and alert users if they try to close a screen with unsaved data.

18. **Make navigation obvious**

    Help users know where they are in the system and how to get where they need to go.

Don'ts

1. Don't leave users wondering if something worked

Whenever a user completes an action like saving a record, sending a message, or submitting a form — give clear, immediate feedback. This can be a success message, a visual change, or even a subtle sound or vibration. Without it, users may repeat actions unnecessarily or assume something went wrong, leading to confusion or duplication.

2. Don't make people wait without explanation

If a system takes time to load or process, show a progress indicator, a loading spinner, or an estimated time to completion. Even a simple "Please wait, this may take a moment" is better than silence. This reassures users that the system hasn't frozen and helps manage their expectations.

3. Don't bury important information

Keep critical details — like patient allergies, appointment times, or urgent alerts — front and centre. Don't hide them behind layers of menus or tabs. Information that's essential for safety, efficiency, or decision-making should always be easy to spot.

4. Don't scare off new users

Complex systems can feel intimidating, especially for newcomers. Keep designs welcoming, clear, and approachable. Use plain language, clear icons, and guided tips or on boarding tours to help new users find their footing without feeling overwhelmed.

5. Don't clutter screens with unnecessary info

Too much information at once can overwhelm users and increase the risk of mistakes. Show only what's needed for the task at hand, and let users drill down for details if they wish. This creates a cleaner, calmer experience and improves focus.

6. Avoid excessive decorative graphics

Design should serve a purpose, not just look pretty. Limit the use of decorative elements that don't help the user achieve their goal. Instead, focus on visuals that support usability, such as clear icons, meaningful illustrations, and helpful diagrams

7. Don't overdo technical jargon

In healthcare, especially language needs to be precise yet understandable. Avoid using overly technical terms or abbreviations in user-facing messages, especially in alerts or error notifications. Plain language builds trust, reduces errors, and improves user satisfaction.

8. Avoid using the same icons for different actions

Icons should act as visual shorthand. If the same symbol is used for multiple, unrelated actions, it creates confusion and undermines trust. Make sure each action has a distinct and recognisable icon and test them with users to ensure clarity.

9. Never use tiny, hard-to-read fonts

Text should be legible across devices and screen sizes. Avoid small fonts, poor contrast, or compressed layouts. Provide adjustable font sizes where possible and follow accessibility standards to ensure readability for users with visual impairments.

10. Don't rely on cryptic icons

A mysterious icon without a label or tooltip forces users to guess its meaning. Stick to widely understood symbols or provide clear labels. For example, a floppy disk icon for "save" may not be meaningful to younger users — a labelled button or modern alternative is often better.

11. Limit abbreviations

Abbreviations can be efficient but also alienating. Only use those that are widely recognised in the healthcare context (like "BP" for blood pressure) and avoid overloading screens with shortened terms that may confuse some users.

12. Don't place dangerous buttons too close together

Accidental taps on the wrong button can have serious consequences. Keep critical actions like "Delete" or "Discharge" separated from routine actions like "Save" or "Next". Consider adding confirmation steps for irreversible actions.

13. Avoid hidden navigation

Don't make users hunt for menus or tools. Make navigation obvious, consistent, and always visible when needed. For example, avoid burying key sections under unfamiliar symbols or gestures, especially on mobile devices.

14. Don't make the help system a maze

When users need help, they're often already frustrated. Make help resources easy to find and navigate, with clear instructions,

FAQs, and contact options. A good help system can be a lifeline; a bad one just adds to frustration.

15. Never risk data loss

In healthcare, data loss can be catastrophic. Implement robust auto save, backup, and recovery mechanisms For example, save drafts of patient notes automatically, and provide clear recovery options if the system crashes or loses connection.

16. Don't make recovery processes mysterious

When something goes wrong, users should know exactly how to fix it. Provide clear, step-by-step guidance on how to recover lost work or resolve an issue. Avoid sending users on a wild goose chase through hidden menus or obscure settings.

17. Avoid making users re-enter the same data

Repetition wastes time and increases the risk of error. Use smart forms, auto fill, and system memory to avoid asking for the same information repeatedly. For example, if a patient's name and date of birth are already in the system, don't ask staff to re-enter them on every screen.

18. Don't leave error messages vague

An error message like "Something went wrong" is frustrating and unhelpful. Explain precisely what happened and how the user can fix it. For example, instead of "Invalid input", say "The date format should be DD/MM/YYYY".

19. Don't let small mistakes pile up

It's better to catch small issues early than to let them escalate. Provide gentle warnings or proactive tips — for example, flagging an incomplete field before submission or reminding users to check for duplicates.

20. Never let critical errors go unchecked

Major errors — like missing mandatory patient data or submitting an incomplete prescription — must be addressed before the user can move on. Require users to fix critical issues immediately, with clear instructions on what's missing or wrong.

At the heart of good UX design for healthcare systems is one simple but powerful idea: respect the user's time, effort, and needs. When we create systems that are clear, supportive, and resilient, we free healthcare professionals to focus on what truly matters and delivering outstanding care to their patients.

Healthcare is a demanding field, often characterised by high pressure, tight timeframes, and life-altering decisions. Every moment a doctor spends wrestling with a cumbersome interface is a moment taken away from patient care. Every confusing error message, every unnecessary click, every lost piece of data adds friction to an already stressful environment. By contrast, well-designed systems act as a silent partner: guiding, assisting, and streamlining processes in the background without drawing attention to themselves.

Good UX in healthcare is not merely about aesthetics or convenience — it's about safety, trust, and well-being. A poorly designed system can lead to medication errors, missed diagnoses, or delays in treatment. A well-designed one can support decision-making, reduce cognitive load, and ensure that the right information reaches the right person at the right time.

Putting People First

Respecting users means understanding who they are and what they need. That includes not only doctors and nurses but also administrative staff, technicians, pharmacists, and sometimes even patients. Each group interacts with the system in different ways and has different priorities — and UX design must cater for all of them.

For example, a nurse on a busy ward may need to access vital signs and medication records quickly and with minimal navigation. A pharmacist may require robust alerts to flag potential drug interactions. Administrative staff may focus on scheduling, billing, and records management. And patients accessing online portals need clear, jargon-free information about their appointments, prescriptions, and test results.

When designing, it's critical to walk in these users' shoes: observe their routines, listen to their frustrations, and test solutions in real-life settings. Design decisions must be driven by empathy, not assumptions.

The Role of Communication and Collaboration

Good UX (User Experience) design doesn't happen in isolation. It thrives in a collaborative environment where designers, developers, clinicians, administrators, and even patients work together. Designers should engage early and often with healthcare professionals — not just at the requirements-gathering stage, but throughout development, testing, and deployment.

Regular feedback loops are essential. A feature that looks brilliant on a whiteboard may stumble in the real world, where hands are gloved, time is short, and attention is divided. Rapid prototyping, usability testing, and iterative improvement are key tools to make sure systems genuinely meet users' needs.

The Importance of Simplicity and Clarity

In the rush to deliver powerful features, it's easy to fall into the trap of complexity. But in healthcare, simplicity is often a life-saver. Cluttered screens, dense menus, and excessive options can overwhelm users and increase the risk of error.

The best systems make complex tasks feel simple. They use clear visual hierarchies, logical layouts, and consistent design patterns to help users navigate confidently. They avoid information overload by focusing on what's essential at each stage of the workflow. They also acknowledge the limits of human attention, offering safeguards like confirmations, error prevention, and undo options.

Designing for Resilience

Healthcare environments are unpredictable. Systems need to be resilient — able to withstand unexpected events without breaking down or losing data. That means designing with contingencies in mind: autosave features to protect work, robust error handling to prevent crashes, and clear recovery paths when something does go wrong.

It also means recognising that no design is perfect on the first try. Healthcare settings evolve, regulations change, and new technologies emerge. UX design must be adaptable, with room for continuous improvement and updates informed by user feedback.

Ethics and Responsibility

With great power comes great responsibility — and nowhere is this more true than in healthcare. UX designers working on healthcare systems are not just building tools; they are shaping experiences that affect people's health, dignity, and sometimes survival.

Ethical considerations must be front and centre. That means protecting patient privacy, ensuring accessibility, and designing systems that are equitable and inclusive. It means resisting the temptation to over-collect data, to lock users into proprietary solutions, or to prioritise efficiency at the expense of empathy.

It also involves balancing automation with human judgement. While decision-support tools can be invaluable, they must be designed as aids, not replacements, for clinical expertise. Users must retain control and be able to override automated recommendations when needed.

Looking Ahead: Innovation and Opportunity

The future of healthcare UX is full of exciting possibilities. Advances in artificial intelligence, wearable technologies, telemedicine, and electronic health records are opening up new ways to improve care. However, innovation must be grounded in human needs.

As we explore voice interfaces, predictive analytics, or personalised dashboards, we must ask: Does this make the clinician's job easier? Does it reduce cognitive burden? Does it help patients feel more in control of their health?

The most successful innovations will be those that put people — not technology — at the centre.

Final Thoughts

Good UX design is often invisible. When it works well, users hardly notice it; they simply get on with their work smoothly and confidently but when it's missing, it's impossible to ignore — errors multiply, frustrations rise, and confidence falters.

Ultimately, designing great healthcare systems is about honouring the trust placed in us by the people on the front lines of care. It's about giving them tools that are not only functional but supportive, respectful, and empowering.

By building systems that respect the user's time, effort, and needs, we help create a healthcare environment where technology lifts burdens rather than adding to them — where clinicians can focus on healing, patients can feel reassured, and the system as a whole moves towards better, safer, and more humane care.

References:

1. Campbell, J. L. (2024). *User experience research and usability of health information technology* (1st ed.). Auerbach Publications. https://doi.org/10.1201/9781003460886

Chapter 05: Scientific Methods of UX Design

Have you ever wondered why, out of dozens of user interface designs submitted by healthcare IT innovators, only one or two are chosen by customers? Often, this happens due to poor communication or the wrong approach to problem-solving. This is where the evolution of UX (User Experience) design methods becomes important.

Traditional UX Design: A Limited Approach

Traditionally, UX design was straightforward. Designers would collect requirements from the customer, come up with a mental plan, and deliver a polished interface. However, the process they used to get there was rarely shared or discussed. This approach focused mainly on producing a solution without properly testing or validating it with the customer during development.

Scientific UX: A Better Way

In contrast, the scientific approach to UX design is more about problem-solving than rushing to a solution. It includes these steps:

1. Clearly define the customer's problem.

2. Create a hypothesis (a possible solution).

3. Test and analyse that solution using real data and feedback.

4. Adjust based on the results and share updates.

5. Repeat the process until the customer is happy.

This method matches well with modern project management styles like Agile and Lean, where collaboration, testing, and constant feedback are key.

Comparing Different Methods of Software Development Methodologies

Waterfall Method

This is the oldest method, where development flows step-by-step, like a waterfall—from planning and design to development, testing, and delivery. It works well when requirements are clear and unlikely to change. However, in fast-moving industries like healthcare IT, customer needs often change. So, waterfall can lead to delays, rework, and frustration when what's delivered doesn't match expectations.

Lean UX

Lean UX is all about "build, measure, and learn." Small cycles (called sprints) are used to create quick sketches or prototypes that are tested by the customer. Because feedback is given regularly, the design can change early before too much time or effort is wasted. This keeps customers involved and helps teams stay on track.

Agile UX

Agile also uses sprints but focuses more on delivering working software at the end of each cycle. It's an engineering-focused process where teams (designers, developers, and product managers) work closely together. Customer feedback happens less frequently than in Lean but is still a part of the process.

Combining Lean and Agile

Combining Lean and Agile gives the best of both worlds. Agile brings structure and working products, while Lean ensures those products match the customer's real needs. Together, they reduce waste, increase speed, and improve product quality.

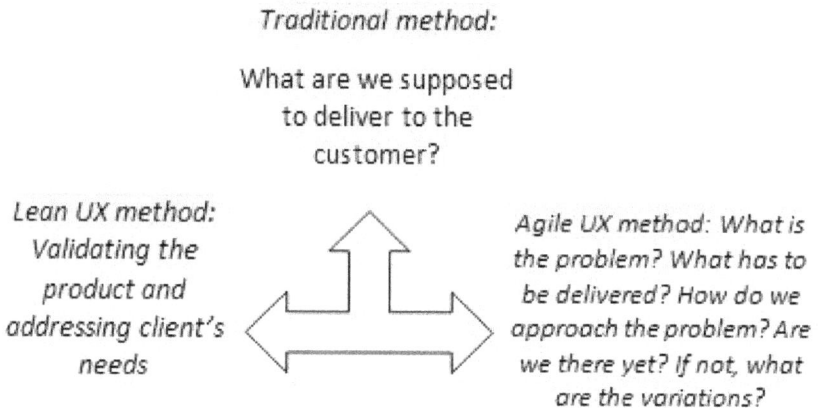

Traditional method:

What are we supposed
to deliver to the
customer?

Lean UX method:
Validating the
product and
addressing client's
needs

Agile UX method: What is
the problem? What has to
be delivered? How do we
approach the problem? Are
we there yet? If not, what
are the variations?

All 3 are different yet share common beliefs

Fictional Use Case Scenarios

1. **Incomplete Communication Example**: A Health IT firm was building a hospital information system. Halfway through development, the team noticed design flaws. They made changes, but this delayed the release. When the final product was delivered, it didn't meet the customer's needs and had technical issues. Only 10% of the staff ended up using it. Why? Because the team didn't follow the Lean principle of building, measuring, and validating at each stage.

2. **Better Communication with Lean+Agile**: In another case, a hospital asked for a new tab in their system to manage chemotherapy prescriptions. Since this impacted many

parts of the system, regular updates and sketches were shared with the client. Internal teams met daily to stay in sync. This kind of active collaboration made sure the final solution was accurate and delivered on time.

3. **Straightforward Case for Waterfall**: A client requested 70 pre-defined reports from a pharmacy system. All the formats and data were specified. Since there was little room for change, the Waterfall or simple Agile method worked fine. In this case, frequent feedback wasn't needed.

Final Thoughts

In today's fast-paced healthcare landscape, where customer needs and regulatory environments are constantly evolving, Health IT companies must adopt development methodologies that prioritize flexibility and efficiency. Approaches like Agile, Lean, or a hybrid of both are increasingly preferred for their ability to deliver the right solutions faster and with minimal waste. While traditional methodologies may still be effective for projects with clearly defined and stable requirements, a Lean-Agile approach is often better suited to real-world scenarios. It empowers teams to adapt quickly, maintain quality, and consistently deliver value that aligns with user expectations.

Comparison of Development Methods in User-Centric Product Design for Health IT			
Methodology	Benefits for User-Centric Product Design	Limitations	Health IT Example

Agile	• Prioritizes features based on user needs • Close collaboration between designers, developers, and stakeholders	• User experience may feel fragmented across sprints • Long-term vision can be hard to maintain	• Enables continuous user feedback and rapid iteration • Prioritizes features based on user needs • Close collaboration between designers, developers, and stakeholders
Lean-Agile (Hybrid)	• Combine Agile speed with Lean efficiency • Maintains focus on user value throughout development • Facilitates both discovery in	• Requires high term maturity and coordination • May become complex without strong leadership	• Developing a clinical support dashboard using dual-track workflows (user research + iterative dev)

	parallel		
Traditional (Waterfall)	• Allows comprehensive design planning upfront • Suitable for projects with fixed compliance requirements • Clear documentation and sign-offs	• Limited ability to adapt to user feedback once development begins • High cost of post-release changes	Building a compliance reporting interface with fixed user requirements and approval-driven workflows

Summary:

- Agile and Lean UX empower user-centric design through early testing and flexibility.

- Lean-Agile Hybrid provides a balanced approach that supports both product discovery and delivery.

- Traditional/Waterfall can be useful where regulatory constraints limit iteration, but risks missing evolving user needs.

References:

1. Gothelf, J., & Seiden, J. (2013). *Lean UX: Applying lean principles to improve user experience*. O'Reilly Media.
2. Beck, K., Beedle, M., van Bennekum, A., Cockburn, A., Cunningham, W., Fowler, M., ... Thomas, D. (2001). *Manifesto for Agile Software Development*. Retrieved from https://agilemanifesto.org/
3. Royce, W. W. (1970). Managing the development of large software systems *Proceedings of IEEE WESCON*, 1–9.

Chapter 6: Does Quality Patient Care Ultimately Rely On Efficiently Designed HIS Interfaces?

You'll be aware by now that Health Information Systems help healthcare professionals take informed clinical decisions and improve quality of patient care.

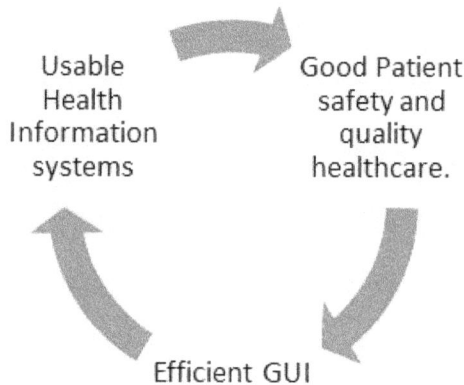

Usable Health Information systems → Good Patient safety and quality healthcare.

Efficient GUI

Consider a system with the following design defects:

1. A health IT system wherein despite the requirement of allergy alert, it is incapable in its design to highlight this to the user. But obviously the end user would miss noticing any allergy alerts, in case the patient has any. Moreover if allergy alerts are related to any drug sensitivity and while prescribing if this is not brought to the notice of the clinician, could be a matter of clinical risk to the patient. Once alerted, the clinician can decide whether to follow it or override the same.

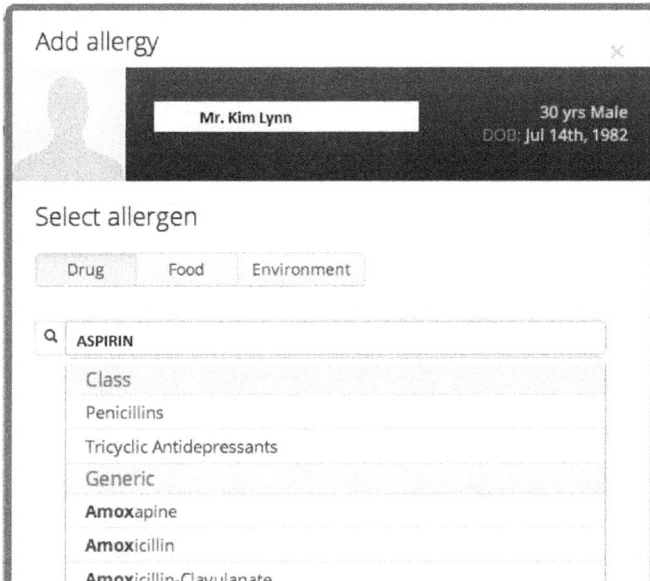

Fig 1.0: Here the allergens are being entered for the patient

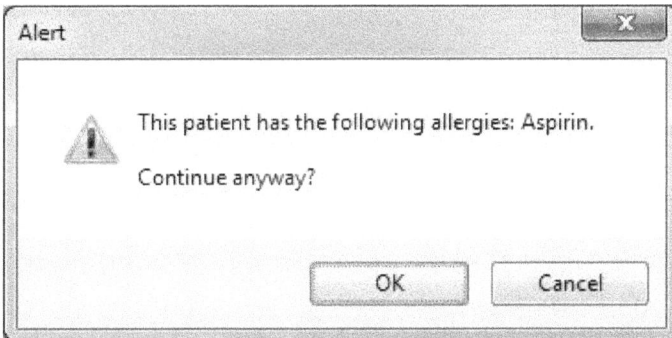

Fig 2.0: Accidentally if one of the allergens (drug) is prescribed, the practitioner is suitably alerted about the same.

2. Assume another example of a Health IT system wherein the design is not effective enough to highlight lab reading differences between a normal and the actual lab test value.

For example the Blood sugar value in the reference range for an adult above 50 years indicates 110 mg/dl as normal, whilst the actual reading taken during the test appears to be 100 mg/dl. Now if the design is incapable of highlighting this difference to the clinician or the concerned lab head, they might miss providing the appropriate treatment to the patient. Eventually the patient's care is at stake.

Section 2 - Lab Test Details

Schedule Date:* Schedule Time: ☐ : ☐ ○ am ○ pm

Lab Test Name	Type	Code	Result	Unit	Normal Range	Abnormal	Location	Remove
Blood Glucose Test	Blood	322		ml	0.0010 - 0.0			☐
Cholera Test	Blood	122.44		ml	5.0 - 15.0			☐

Remove

Fig 3.0: The lab results are entered for their actual result value along with the normal and above normal ranges, one way of alerting the practitioner

VetLyte® Electrolyte Analyzer			11/11/2008 8:00:00 PM
CL	100 mmol/L	112 - 129	
K	3 mmol/L	3.6 - 5.8	
NA	160 mmol/L	150 - 165	

VetTest® Chemistry Analyzer			11/11/2008
ALKP	79.7 U/L	23 - 212	
ALT	50 U/L	10 - 100	
BUN	20 mg/dL	7 - 27	
CREA	0.89 mg/dL	0.5 - 1.8	
GLU	96 mg/dL	77 - 125	
TP	6.1 g/dL	4.8 - 7	

1   2   3   4

Fig 4.0: Here 1   represents the analyte; 2 result value; 3 Reference range; 4   tabular format of results. Green   Normal range; Blue   below normal range; Red   Above normal range. This could be another way of representing the lab results with suitable colour indicators to alert the user.

3. Consider an example wherein the Pharmacist allocates (keeps them ready) the required medications to several patients. The design of the system is such that at this stage of allocation the pharmacist can generate relevant patient leaflet (containing details of the medication for patient education) and this patient leaflet is now stored which can be retrieved at the final or the dispensing phase. At the dispensing stage the patient is physically handed over their medications and the pharmacist now retrieves the patient leaflets using a dropdown menu. This dropdown menu contains only the Patient IDs of those patients to whom the medications have been physically handed over. Now with such a design there is a probability that :

   a. The pharmacist can select the wrong patient ID, become confused, and provide the wrong patient leaflet. This would be when the patients don't recollect their own ID, it becomes more difficult to retrieve information rather becomes a lengthy process to archive the information.
   b. Or on the other hand if using the dropdown option, the patient ID of those patients to whom the leaflet has been dispatched should not appear in the dropdown menu during the next action. However again the possibility of not recollecting the patient ID could be a concern.
   c. Ideally at the time of handing over the printed patient leaflets at the dispensing stage Patient names along with Patient IDs could be displayed.

Even after considering the above options, providing dropdown menus to retrieve any patient related information in general is clinically risky as it can lead to high frequency of errors. In the above example, it can be a huge patient ID list. It will be practically impossible for the pharmacist to go through this long list of even 100 or 200 IDs despite providing patient names. Rather it would be ideal to generate the leaflet while the allocation step itself here in this above example and hand the printed patient leaflet (hard copy) at the dispensing stage to avoid any confusion. Again you may want to argue about providing dropdown menus to set controlled values (a list that has definite values) such as a set of drugs allergic to or food allergic towards, recorded against the patient. However an uncontrolled list such names of countries or patient IDs, which are not constant and keep changing frequently, would be rather cumbersome to operate using drop-down menus. Please refer to figs 5.0 and 6.0 below.

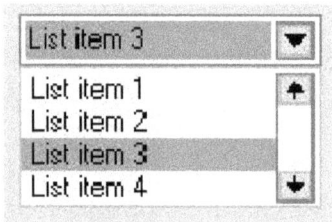
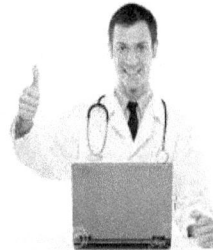

Fig 5.0

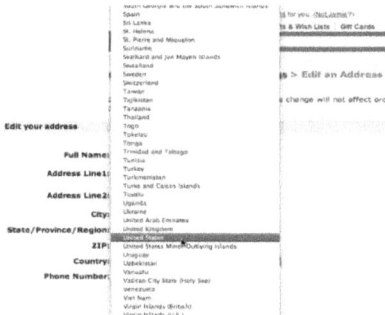
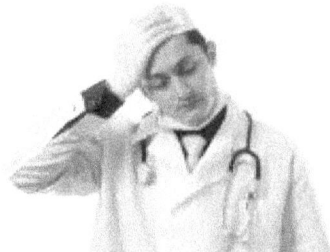

Fig 6.0

Hence as seen from the above instances it is the effective and safer IT design that will ensure development of safer Health IT products and in turn promote safe patient care. Hence Health IT product design is a shared responsibility among developers, implementers, and users across the various stages of the health IT life cycle, which include design and development; implementation and customisation; upgrades, maintenance, and operations; and risk identification, mitigation, and remediation. Following security and privacy guidelines also form a part of providing patient safety through efficient GUI, which shall be discussed in a separate section. Another way to ensure safer design of Health IT products is to check on the regulatory aspects and the interoperability and exchange of information across health systems This eventually calls for verifying the quality of data that resides in these Health IT products.

The fact that Health IT systems are used to make informed clinical decisions but cannot replace the existing clinical decision making capabilities of the clinician should be considered. A way to assure that this safety is built into the health IT system is to include this kind of a safety check right from the start that is the requirement specification stage. Business analysts and Health IT designers can brainstorm right at this beginning stage to categorize requirements according to the potential clinical risks that such requirements would pose. The team can then decide on the effective design to achieve that requirement.

Chapter 7: Few Myths and Realities of Health IT Systems

Like in any other domain, Myths, half-truths, realities do persist in Health IT as well. In this chapter let's discuss few myths and realities of Health IT systems and never know you may also stumble across various myths that you believed to be true:

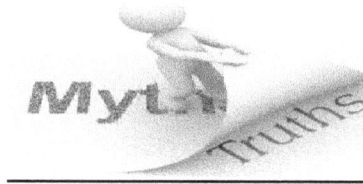

Myth #1: **Usability of Health IT systems is affected only by the software design**

Reality: Not only does design implicate the usability of a system, but the amount of training imparted to the user during implementation of a system also affects the usability. For instance if the end user is imparted with inaccurate or incomplete knowledge about the use of the system, they would not be in a position to use it effectively to their fullest of potential. Likewise when the workflows itself is incorrectly understood and passed on to the design team, no matter how effective the deign if the workflow is incorrect or does not fit the requirements of the end user still usability of the system will remain a concern.

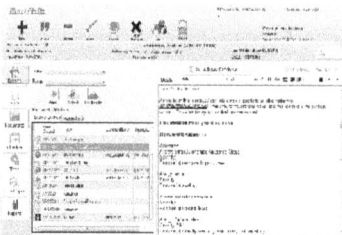

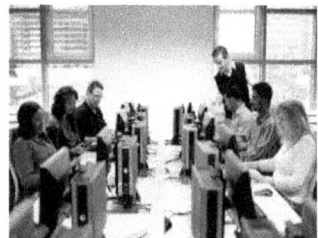

95

Software design Vs HIS training

Myth#2: Making software screens and layouts simple, and providing a good font size throughout with a good colour standardization, will make a system usable.

Reality: Though good colour standardization, visibility, font size and simple layouts are important, focusing only on these will not be sufficient. Rather it is the content that goes in such designs that matters. Ultimately it is the content that has to effectively stored, archived and retrieved by the clinician to make informed clinical decisions. Hence a good design should support a smooth mechanism to such data or content

E- abilities of Health IT Systems Vs relevant Content flow

Myth#3: Good usable systems should be user centric, give users want they want or demand

Reality: Often what the users demand could be wrong or their requirements could pose a clinical risk to the product. Hence the product team should perform an evidence based research of similar available features and decide whether it is clinically and technically correct to provide such a feature as requested by the end user.

User requirements/ideas Vs Relevant usable system set for a purpose

Myth#4: Intuitive Health IT systems such as those with good design require no training

Reality: Since Healthcare data is complex, no matter how intuitive the design, it is still important to impart proper training while implementation. With proper training the user's competency and in turn the systems competency can be measured. This can further help to revise the product for betterment.

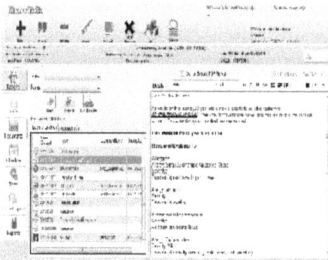

Don't get bogged down with your medical facility EMRs

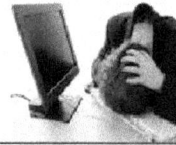

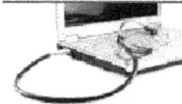

Healthcare data is complex, we're there to help, please undergo training.

Thoughtfully designed systems Vs User training

To summarize, a good design is essential to develop an intuitive Health IT product, which will help the clinician to make informed medical decisions, and provide quality care to the patients. This is in turn achieved only by imparting proper training of the product to the clinician. Eventually the clinician's ease to use the product will help to assess the usability of the system.

Chapter 8: Security -Privacy concerns and Usable HIS

What is Security in Healthcare?

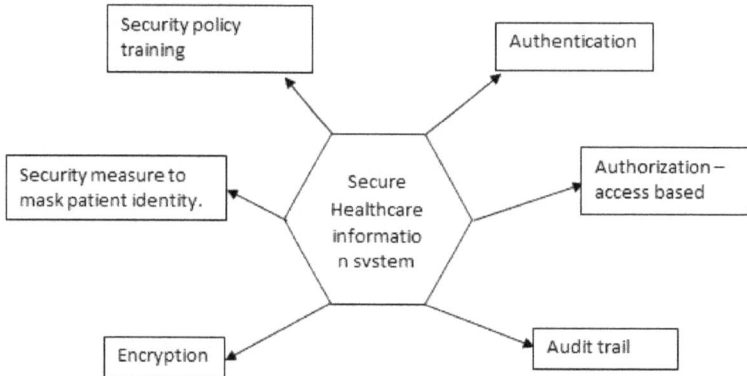

Security policy training

Authentication

Security measure to mask patient identity.

Secure Healthcare informatio n svstem

Authorization – access based

Encryption

Audit trail

What is Health information security and why is this important to manage health data?

It's a moral and ethical responsibility of healthcare organisations to safeguard sensitive information of their patients and employees. Security is just such an administrative and technical procedure put in place to ensure secured health information. When it comes to handling complex and private health records in EHR it is utmost priority to ensure that the system has distinct technical as well as graphical interface features to protect data vulnerability.

Access control is one of the key security feature consideration to protect privacy of health information. Access control can be achieved by the following thoughts:

Confidentiality: That patient health records are not made available or disclosed to any unauthorized individual

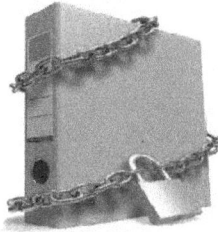

Your health information is safe with us. Here patient privacy is considered.

Integrity: That patient health data cannot be altered nor destroyed in an unauthorized manner

With security features in place data integrity is intact.

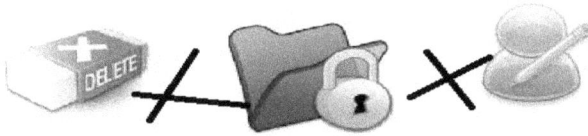

Availability: That patient information is made available for sharing with authorised users in an authorised manner.

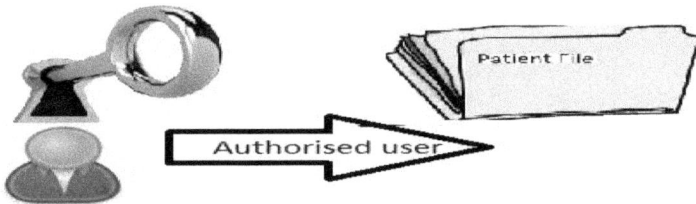

What is Privacy in Healthcare?

Privacy in Healthcare organisations is the right of the patient to keep their medical records in private free from the threat of being disclosed to others.

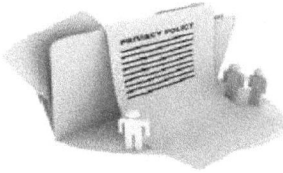

Please respect my right to holding my records in secret.

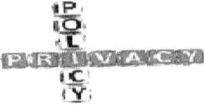

Confidentiality is the communication between two parties, in this case the Health facility and the patient such that a commitment is made by the health facility to the patients that their information would not be disclosed without proper authorisation. Security is a mechanism in place through technical and graphical interface to assure this confidentiality policy is taken care of considering the patient privacy.

<u>**Relationship between the two**</u>

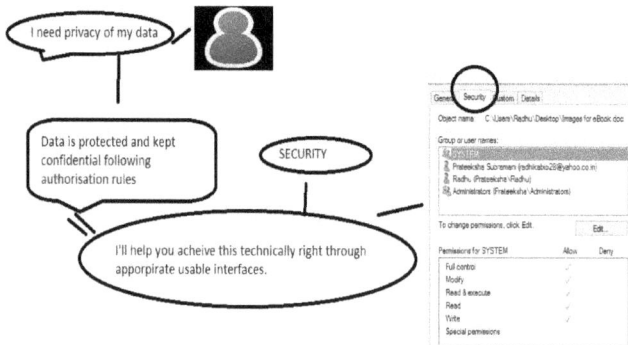

Privacy and security are quite different from each other. Privacy is a legal or ethical concern wherein the patient seeks right to hold his/her information confidentially. Whereas security is a technical thingy wherein appropriate at the front-end and the back-end of the system to ensure privacy concern is taken care of. In short security process is to be implemented to ensure privacy as the end consequence. There are many proposed privacy laws HIPPA privacy being one of them. Security with respect to these would mean to have those procedures and structures in place to maintain confidentiality in order to abide by such privacy laws to avoid breach of the law.

A quick revamp:

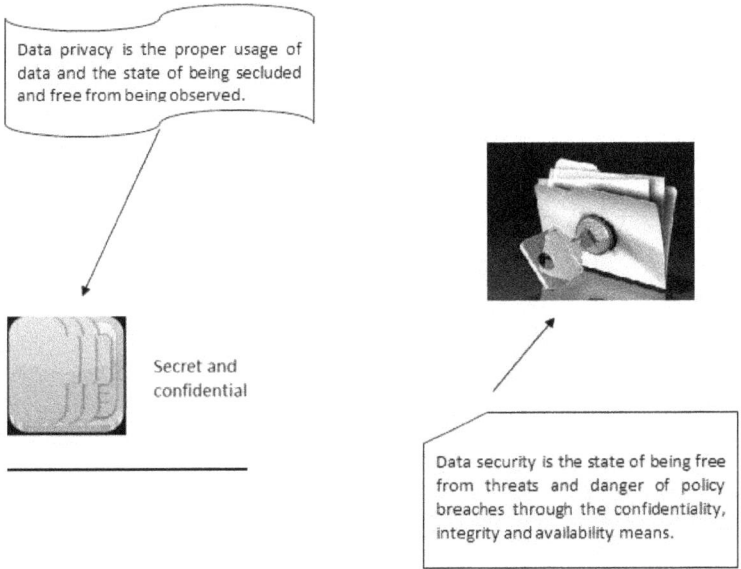

Data privacy is the proper usage of data and the state of being secluded and free from being observed.

Secret and confidential

Data security is the state of being free from threats and danger of policy breaches through the confidentiality, integrity and availability means.

There may be number of reasons for misusing a patient's health records. These could be intentional or unintentional resulting into breaching of patient data confidently.

Example: *Assume that during the patient's admission into the hospital if they befriend one of the health care staff may be a nurse or a doctor or any person from the administrative department. Now after the patient is discharged from the hospital, what if somehow the friend (may be a nurse, doctor) tries to fetch the contact details of the patient by accessing his/her health records. Again there may be possibilities without the consent of the clinician in-charge of the treating the patient, the patient records are used for clinical research purposes by the clinical team of the hospital. This is again another ethical breach.*

Earlier with paper based records the only means of securing information would be to either lock the relevant documents in a safe place or inform only the authorised person about the documents. So it was just lock and key to ensure security of patient information However with the invention of electronic records, there is definitely more scope to improve the way patient information is stored, archived and shared in an authorised manner. Moreover with many patient data protection acts in place the concern of patient data confidentiality is definitely taken care of.

Few prominent such patient confidentiality acts are Computer misuse act 1990, Access to Health records act 1990, The Data protection act 1998 and Freedom of information act of 2000. Few principles in common, with any such protection acts are that:

- o Only limited patient information should be processed for the required purpose

- o What, how, where and when the health information should be shared has to be decided with the patient's consent

- o The patient information should be stored in a secure manner (by defining the relevant access controls) and should be available to the concerned person upon demand.

- o Every patient information should be defined with a shelf life. No health information of any patient should be stored longer than it is required. A definite period for either deactivation, suspension or termination of the patient health record should be appropriately defined.

Just as how the clinicians should have rights to access and share their patient health records with other fellow physicians, it is equally important that the patient should also have the rights to determine what, how, to whom, where and when their health information should be shared.

HIPAA privacy rules

With electronic health records, the concern of patient data confidentiality and security has gained more importance. HIPPA (Health insurance portability and accountability) act 1996 defines policies and procedures for standardisation of electronic health records and thus considering the breach of patient confidentiality and integrity of data, ensuring sharing of health information data of the patient in a secured and authorised manner. HIPPA requires that patient health information recorded by the health care provider like notes, observations or any medical history should not be disclosed for any other purposes other than treatment, payment and other health care operations included in the HIPPA act.

Two main HIPPA privacy rules regarding the patient treatment is as follows:

- o HIPPA privacy rules prohibits the sharing of patient information by the health care provider with any of their health facility employees including fellow colleagues involved with the treatment, without the patient's written letter of authorisation.

- o The HIPPA privacy rule encourages the communication between the patient and the health care providers involved in the patient's treatment, using emails. However appropriate safeguards should be ensured whist communication of patient health information via email such that there is threat to the integrity and confidentiality to the patient data.

  - o Furthermore to ensure integrity and confidentiality of the patient health information, HIPPA mandates health facilities to conduct audit trails, to identify as to who should have access to the patient health information. As per HIPPA rules, audit logs can be maintained up to 6 years.

As seen above with concerns revolving around the confidentiality, security and integrity and availability of patient information, it is essential that electronic Health Information Systems have the provision to address these concerns with an *effective GUI*.

Is your HIS HIPAA compliant?

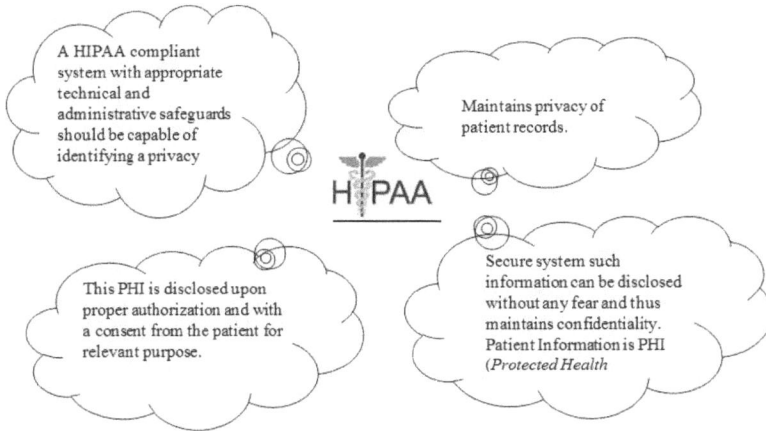

A HIPAA compliant system with appropriate technical and administrative safeguards should be capable of identifying a privacy

Maintains privacy of patient records.

H PAA

This PHI is disclosed upon proper authorization and with a consent from the patient for relevant purpose.

Secure system such information can be disclosed without any fear and thus maintains confidentiality. Patient Information is PHI (*Protected Health*

Security with effective GUI; Use case scenarios:

As seen above, patient data confidentiality is indeed a subject that needs careful consideration while dealing with electronic health records. This can be achieved by designing UIs that provide the appropriate access control mechanisms to assure that privilege to access patient data is provided in an authorised manner to only the authorized people. Assigning the pertinent action control functions like EDIT, ADD, MODIFY and DELETE to the concerned person is also essential.

Patients have the right to determine when, how and to what extent their health information should be shared by their clinician with other health care professionals who are involved in the treatment of the patient. AN effective GUI should help achieve this.

Example: *consider a patient management system, wherein the clinician has recorded certain health information about the patient in terms of their allergy, medical history details, laboratory results, X-ray, scan images and details of certain medications (especially controlled or scheduled drugs). Now for some reason the clinician would want to share few important health information of this* *patient with their fellow clinicians just to have a second opinion on the treatment to be offered to the patient. In such case, there should be a GUI wherein the patient should have an option to give privilege either to 'VIEW ONLY', or 'EDIT and 'VIEW', or 'ADD, EDIT and VIEW' to only those relevant healthcare professionals (users) who are involved in the treatment of the patient.*

Let's consider few case studies here as a basis to understand how effective GUIs could be designed to ensure security, confidentiality and integrity of patient data.

Case study 1: Patient confidentiality

Assume that Endocrinologist Dr Saraha's best friend Mary pays visit to the same hospital where Dr Sarah work. Mary is asked to consult the gynaecologist Dr Gomes. Dr Gomes and Dr Sarah are again best colleagues as they work in the same health facility. Whilst consultation the following information about Mary were recorded by Dr Gomes:

1. Demographic details

2. Prenatal examination records

   • Medications

   • Scans

   • Blood tests

3. Follow-up consultation details.

Dr Gomes and Dr Sarah share the same desktop for accessing relevant information of the patients, but with different passwords. Mary and Dr Sarah have a brief chat. For some reason Dr Sarah is eager to know the reason for Mary's visit. Dr Sarah tries to retrieve the demographic details of Mary from the common patient records. However access to the medical records of Mary is denied to Dr Sarah. The system requests to enter a username and password to access the record.

Design wise, an access control was set at the parameter level itself by the administrator such that patient information recorded by Dr Gomes is not accessible to any other fellow clinicians, without the authorised consent of Dr Gomes. Hence Mary's health data was not accessible to Dr Sarah.

Case study 1a: Dr Gomes first takes a written consent from Mary requesting Mary to allow Dr Gomes to share her health information with Dr Sarah, who will be involved in her treatment as well. After Mary's written consent, Dr Gomes requests the administrator to give a 'READ' only access to Dr Sarah with a unique username and password to access Mary's information for a set period of time. The parameters thus defined here are:

User: Dr Sarah; Permission: VIEW only; time limit: 3 months (calendar setting).

Case study 1b: Dr Sarah is an endocrinologist. Mary is 6 weeks and is advised by Dr Gomes to get her Thyroid levels checked. The laboratory results show high levels of T3 and T4 which were not safe for pregnancy. Hence Dr Gomes advises Mary to consult Dr Sarah. Dr Sarah advises Mary to take Thyroxin medicines to bring down the levels of T3 and T4. Mary informs Dr Gomes and corresponding information is entered into Mary's patient records. Now with Mary's written consent, Dr Gomes gives Dr Sarah a 'READ' and 'ADD' access without any permission to edit the existing data. Thus Dr Sarah can also add Mary's medical information pertaining to her department, so that Mary's complete pre-natal treatment history is available in a single system file.

The permissions defined by the administrator are:

User: Dr Sarah; Access: READ and ADD. Time -limit: 3 months.

Patient Confidentiality Use case scenarios:

Patient confidentiality as seen above is a principle within medical ethics specified even in Dorland's medical dictionary. It states it as the ethical and moral responsibility of both the healthcare provider and the facility to not disclose the patient health information in an unauthorised manner.

With paper records earlier few healthcare providers were of the opinion that it was much simpler to avoid any confidentiality breach. However one may also want to argue that rather with Electronic health records system though technically challenging but is much simpler to protect confidentiality and patient privacy than paper records where data breach vulnerability is more, due to less stringent security control.

Before we start with the use case scenarios with respect to what the GUIs should provide in terms of securing patient confidentiality, let's look at what information/medical cases should be kept confidential.

Medical Information that can be kept confidential:

1. **Patient Identity:** This is relevant wherein either a celebrity, member of a royal family or a VIP pays a visit to the hospital and would not want to reveal their identity.

2. **Clinical information:** Certain clinical information in certain countries that could create a stigma, such as:

- Patient diagnosed with HIV or other communicable disease

- Unmarried lady diagnosed with pregnancy

- Revealing the sex of the foetus (in certain countries)

- Unmarried or married women undergone Dilatation and Curettage.

- Medical examination of rape victims

- Patients undergoing Psychiatric treatments

Certain circumstances where confidentiality could be compromised:

1. When a to-be couple come in for a HIV test, and the male is tested positive for HIV. The health counsellor cannot avoid but tell the female that she could also pose a risk if she plans to marry. Moreover it's the ethical and moral duty of the healthcare counsellor to provide this information to the female despite the male's consent to not disclose the information. One may want to argue this kind of a confidentiality breach as either good or bad? Or how could the EHR be designed such that this moral responsibility is not considered as a breach of confidentiality?

2. Clinical research institutions: Here the patient undergoing treatment in a medical institution should imply that they have no objection of their data being used for clinical research purposes. Nonetheless patient consent is required. However by virtue it being a medical institution can they let go this authorisation process and still use the

patient data for medical research purpose? Can this be a confidentiality breach? Is confidentiality compromised in here?

3. A case wherein a schizophrenic patient is posing a life threating risk to other patient due to his sudden violent behaviour. In this case to bring the condition under control it is essential to let other senior practitioners and the family members know this situation. Again a situation which is neither under the control of the healthcare staff nor the facility and will this result to a breach?

4. In case of Medico legal case or a general report to the local health department on communicable diseases, report on usage of narcotic drugs again patient confidentiality could be compromised.

<u>GUI functions to aid in protecting patient confidentiality:</u>

1. To protect patient identity provision to generate an 'Alias name' can be provided.

    a. **Use case scenario**: *A Hollywood celebrity gets herself registered in a private health facility for a minor cosmetic surgery. The registration is carried out by a senior authority Mr Mark in the facility to whom the administrator has given access to register this patient with an 'Alias' and the 'Real' name. Mr Mark has full access as to 'Add', 'Edit', 'Modify', 'Delete' and 'View' details of this Hollywood actress. He has assigned 'Add', 'Edit' and 'View Only' access to two more practitioners Dr Jones and Dr Williams in-charge of this minor surgery. Hence when the medical records of this patient is opened by Dr Jones and Williams of the 'Cosmetology' department the patient records are* *available for entering new data, editing the entered data and for viewing. However they are neither able to modify the earlier details such as the registration details entered by registration front desk officer Mr Mark nor able to delete the same. Apart from this the record of this patient is tagged for confidentiality and not available to any other practitioners in the cosmetology department and the record is inactive or as if doesn't exist for view to rest of the department.*

2. Only authorised users of the health facility should be given the access control to register the patient by both 'Alias' as well as 'Real name'.

    a. **Use case scenario**: *The Hollywood actress returns for a follow-up with Dr Jones, after two weeks of the surgery. Mr Mark had marked the confidentiality status for this patients for a period of 6 months. Now since Dr Jones has the privilege to add, edit and view the records of this patient, he tries opening the chart. The system populates a screen prompting for the username and password, Dr Jones enters the relevant details and the patient summary chart is available to him for further system operation.*

3. A parameter at the administrative level in the GUI should be such that the registration record of this patient should be available for add, edit, modify, view and delete only to the authorised user. The registration details of this patient should be hidden for the other users or should be in a disabled mode.

4. For any operation such as 'add, edit, modify, delete or view the system should populate a screen for the authorised users to enter their username and password

and upon retrieving the correct password should allow this user to perform the functions.

5. There should be a parameter such that the authorised user can generate relevant reports using the 'Alias' as well as the 'real name' of the patient.

    a. **Use case scenario:** *The local health department of a certain state in North America requests for a monthly report on the usage of narcotic drugs in its pharmacy department. Amber health facility is one which comes under this province. The report format reads as:*

    i. *Date; Department; Doctor-in charge; Patient; Dose details; purpose; witness; remarks. Here Mr Mark has the privilege to access records of all patients that are tagged for the confidentiality status. He then generates the report in the above format and in this process retrieves records of two patients that are marked as confidential for the usage of Morphine. He then retrieves the real name as well and generates the above report in both alias and real name.*

6. Audit trail should be maintained to record the transactions carried out using both the alias and the real name.

7. There could be a time parameter set at the facility level to maintain the confidentiality status of the patient. In short the confidentiality status could be activated and deactivated for a certain time frame depending on the need.

8. To maintain patient confidentiality tag whenever the user logs off and wants to login the system should populate a

screen asking the user to enter the username and password again within a time frame.

9. There could be a screen wherein the authorised personnel could define access privilege for other users who can perform certain set of functions on the record that has been marked as confidential. Again the user can give privilege to other users to perform these functions only on certain set of records such as either only on the registration details or on the clinical data and so on.

10. There could be provision to set a confidentiality tag at various levels such as only at the patient registration stage, Medical records pertaining to all or specific encounters, or entirely at a specific department level.

   a.   15 yrs old Ms Celina with the complaint of Amenorrhoea for the past two months books an appointment with the gynaecologist Dr Linda of the Amber healthcare facility. Dr Linda requests Celina to undertake yet another urine test and also suggests for a blood test. The results turned out to be positive. Ms Celina requests for another appointment with Dr Linda after two weeks. Upon reading the lab results and considering this as a sensitive case Dr Linda marks this 2nd encounter with Celina as confidential and this record now is available only to Dr Linda.

   i. After a couple of weeks Ms Celina complains of severe abdominal pain. However Dr Linda is on a vacation and the only gynaecologist available that day was Dr Deann. Celina confirms her appointment with Dr Deann with no other option but to get cured from the abdominal pain. Dr Deann *tries to refer to the details of the first encounter and is able to view the details. Going further when Dr Deann tries to open the patient records of the 2nd encounter, she is prompted by the system to enter a username and password, as this particular encounter was tagged confidential by Dr Linda. Since Dr Deann is unaware of the relevant username and password she is unable to access the records.*

11. Again to re ascertain confidentiality there could be a periodic change of passwords and after consecutive three failed attempts the access should be denied.

12. Biometrics can be used to provide authentication.

13. Overriding privileges to higher authorities to unmask the confidentiality tag should be provided in case of emergencies and other medical situations.

   a.   ***Use case scenario***: *53yr old Mr Porter is a schizophrenic patient. He is admitted to the ER department for immediate attention due to history of aggression since last night. After physical assessment by Dr Hick it was diagnosed that Mr Porter's condition is severe and threating to other patients in the ward. Dr Hick learns from Porter's family that he had been here a month ago for a brief check-up with Dr Crowther. Dr Crowther had then tagged the patient records as confidential. Hence when Dr Hick tries to open the previous encounter history of Mr Porter, the system prompts for a username and password, which Dr Hick is unaware of. This being a case of emergency, the senior authority requests the administrator Mr Mark to grant Dr Hick a special access to Porter's* *previous records for a time period of 2 days. Dr Hick now has full access to the records of this patient for 2 days.*

14. Encryption can be used while exchanging emails of such patient records.

References

1. Basil, N. N., Akpan, F., & Basil, H. U. (2022). Health Records Database and Inherent Security Concerns. Frontiers in Health Informatics, 11(2), 134–147. https://www.ncbi.nlm.nih.gov/pmc/articles/PMC9647912/
2. Theodos, K., & Zucker, J. (2020). Health Information Privacy Laws in the Digital Age: HIPAA and Beyond. Missouri Medicine, 117(6), 567–573. https://www.ncbi.nlm.nih.gov/pmc/articles/PMC7883355/
3. Edemekong, P. F., Haydel, M. J., & Singh, S. (2024). Health Insurance Portability and Accountability Act (HIPAA). In StatPearls. StatPearls Publishing. https://www.ncbi.nlm.nih.gov/books/NBK500019/

Chapter 9: Positive Psychology and UX Design

Principles of positive psychology could be applied to UX design in healthcare technology to enhance engagement and user experience. By emphasizing factors such as meaningful interactions, motivation, and satisfaction, these principles can help create digital environments that support both clinicians and patients. For clinicians, this might involve streamlined workflows, reduced cognitive load, and interfaces that facilitate efficient decision-making. For patients, it could include intuitive navigation, clear communication of health information, and features that encourage active participation in their care. Overall, integrating positive psychology into healthcare UX has the potential to improve usability while fostering a sense of involvement, empowerment, and engagement across all users.

Positive psychology, though formally established in 1998 by Dr Martin Seligman, has roots in earlier contributions from William James and Abraham Maslow, who laid the groundwork by emphasizing human potential, personal growth, and well-being (James, 2018; Maslow, 2006). This evolving field gained momentum as it transitioned from treating mental illness to focusing on factors that help individuals flourish, culminating in Seligman's PERMA model, which underscores Positive Emotions, Engagement, Relationships, Meaning, and Achievement as central to well-being(Seligman, 2011). "Meaning," in particular, is highlighted for its profound influence on motivation, purpose, and satisfaction in both personal and professional contexts. Viktor Frankl's Man's Search for Meaning (Frankl, 2008) emphasizes the vital importance of finding purpose, especially during difficult times, noting that "those who have a 'why' to live can bear almost any 'how.'" This highlights the essential role of meaning for professionals, as history demonstrates that it is crucial for both personal and professional fulfilment, and in today's context is even more important in fields like healthcare.

In healthcare, the rapid evolution of digital health tools, such as electronic health records and telemedicine, has not only bought significant advancements but also introduced challenges like developer burnout and dissatisfaction (Evans, 2016; Mellblom et al., 2019). Studies show that many healthcare software developers face high turnover rates and decreased productivity, often due to burnout and a lack of purpose in their work (Trinkenreich et al., 2023). Burnout, characterized by emotional exhaustion, depersonalization, and limitation of personal accomplishments, has been an identified problem since the late 20th century (Mellblom et al., 2019). It was found out through a survey by Haystack Analytics[1] about 80 – 83% of software developers from different groups face burnout, job dissatisfaction, and a high turnover rate. According to the 2021, Bureau of Labor Statistics[2] software developers have an average turnover rate of 57.3%. The study also reveals that 29% of these departures were involuntary, while 25% were voluntary.

Burnout among developers in healthcare software will limit the adoption and effectiveness of technology because high levels of stress and dissatisfaction can be easily related to a lack of motivation and low productivity. Burnout results in a reduction of productivity among workers in the tech industry (Tulili et al., 2023). High levels of stress and burnout along with a lost sense of purpose and meaning in developers could impede such a lack of understanding and impact the adoption of technology.

While the intervention of technology in healthcare has significantly improved clinical and patient outcomes, the well-being of healthcare technology professionals has emerged as a critical concern (Graziotin et al., 2018). Where there has been progress in the adoption of healthcare technologies and other wearable devices, the adoption rate is never even. For instance, according to research [1] a lack of understanding among software developers about healthcare practices and workflows contributes significantly as one of the barriers faced in the adoption of information technology in healthcare. This gap in understanding can lead to poorly designed systems that do not meet the needs of healthcare providers, ultimately affecting patient care.

Even though, several mobile health apps and EHRs have been created to help healthcare providers to actively enter the patient's data, archive it and interpret it but their lack of accessibility at the right time and in the right manner causes delays and severely affects the patient's health. In the era of fast-paced technology these issues remain unresolved.

Usability and Its Importance in Digital Health Technologies

We have seen the various forms of complex health data that must be managed appropriately within healthcare technology to make informed decisions. Beyond institutional systems, there is vast data available on personal health — from diabetes self-management to post-operative chemotherapy care, hypertension management at home, and more.

Whether it is a hospital information system relevant to professionals or health awareness information for individuals, several usability questions arise:

1. Does a hospital information product (EHR, EMR, PHR, mobile medical app, or health website) display information in an intuitive manner?

2. Is the user able to interpret the relevant message from the screens displayed? In hospital systems, are relevant alerts and messages prompted?

3. Can the user browse for desired information promptly?

4. Can the user navigate smoothly from one information set to another in a meaningful flow?

5. Is the user alerted about important information, with options to rectify errors?

Accessibility, understanding and interpretation of healthcare solution is crucially important and this is where the digital health tools become unstable causing further complications for healthcare providers and delays in immediate response to patient's health.

To support designers in creating healthcare technologies that foster engagement and meaningful user experiences, platforms like PERMA Integrated Health provide insightful articles and resources. Many designers struggle with translating theoretical concepts, such as positive psychology, into practical UX solutions that work for both clinicians and patients. Our blog addresses this challenge by offering evidence-based guidance, case studies, and practical strategies to help designers understand user needs, promote engagement, and design interfaces that enhance the overall healthcare experience. By bridging the gap between theory and practice, these resources empower designers to create technology that is not only usable but also contributes to well-being and meaningful interactions.

This approach emphasizes Positive emotions, Engagement, Relationships, Meaning, and Accomplishments in designing digital health tools, ensuring that technology contributes positively to both professional workflows and patient experiences. Looking ahead, a dedicated edition will focus exclusively on applying the PERMA framework to healthcare UX, providing designers with deeper insights and actionable strategies to integrate well-being into every aspect of health technology design.

What is Usability?
According to the International Organization for Standardization (ISO), usability is *"the effectiveness, efficiency, and satisfaction with which intended users can achieve their tasks in the intended context of product use."*

1. **Effectiveness:** the degree to which the interface facilitates task completion.

2. **Efficiency:** the time taken to complete a task.

3. **Satisfaction:** the user's subjective sense of ease and comfort.

Other definitions, such as Preece et al. (1994), highlight learnability, safety, effectiveness, and efficiency. The NCCD further frames usability through TURF (Task, User, Representation, and Function).https://sbmi.uth.edu/nccd/ehrusability/evaluation/turf/

The TURF framework consists of:

1. **Useful:** Does the healthcare system support users with sufficient domain content and relevant workflows?

2. **Usable:** is the system user friendly and errorless?

3. **Learnability:** how immediate is its response to the given task?

4. **Efficiency:** how quickly it accomplishes a task?

5. **Error tolerance:** does it correct and help users avoid mistakes?

In sum, usability is not merely "look and feel," but whether systems function in a way that is genuinely easy to use.

Hypothetical Case Studies: Usability Nightmares in Health IT
Case Study 1: *A Cardiologist's Frustration*

Mrs. Kerry Smith, aged 36, was rushed to A\&E with stabbing chest pain. Initial ECG and blood pressure readings appeared normal. Dr Ray, a cardiologist, was consulted, and further tests were ordered, including a chest X-ray. The X-ray was uploaded into the system, and Dr Ray accessed it remotely via his mobile app. However, the small screen size, font size, and low contrast ratio of the app made interpretation impossible. This led to unnecessary repeat tests (ECG, ECHO, bloodwork). Ultimately, the problem was usability, not medical expertise.

This case shows how bad usability in mobile health apps can cause clinical delays, repeated testing, and unnecessary patient stress.

Case Study 2: *Paediatric Prescribing App*

A paediatrician uses a prescribing app with an in-built calculator. Fields such as age and weight were not marked as mandatory, meaning the app could generate a default dose without them. Its wrong interpretation can cause severe damage and threaten a patient's life, for instance if it prescribes the same medicine dosage for a child weighing 22 pounds and a child weighing 44 pounds-this could be fatal!

Additionally, if the app took two minutes to calculate dosages during an emergency, it would be unusable in urgent care. Here, poor usability (mandatory fields, calculation speed) translates into serious clinical risk.

Reflecting on the Consequences of Bad Usability

Bad usability in health IT is not just inconvenient; it can be dangerous. Consider medication administration or laboratory systems. If the system fails to clearly highlight the abnormality in a patient's blood glucose level, the clinician might interpret it as normal and cause further threat to the patient's life at that urgent moment.

To help ensure the thumb rule of healthcare is followed, collaboration between Positive Psychology (PERMA) to healthcare technology is the solution. This framework — PERMA ((Positive Emotion, Engagement, Relationships, Meaning, Accomplishment) — helps to make sure systems are functional and improves professional well-being.

Positive Emotion: user friendly design, soothing tone, gamification → reduces frustration.

Engagement: optimize process, less distractions → increased concentration & productivity.

Relationships: socially engaging tasks, team-centred tools → improvement in interpersonal relations and strong teamwork.

Meaning: effects of impact clearly displayed on dashboards →
easy access, less burnout.

Accomplishment: indicates progress, provides feedback →
reinforcing & efficient.

Implementation strategy:

> 1. Engaging features for healthcare professionals.
>
> 2. Multi-disciplinary approach (designers, behavioural
> scientists, clinicians).
>
> 3. Continuous evaluation of its usage & improved results.

Conclusion

Poor access and lagging of patients' sensitive health information
on the healthcare technology causes frustration and harms
patients, especially at critical moment. Embedding of positive
psychology to UX design has helped solved this issue and it not
only takes care of health-related issues but also addresses their
emotional needs. This leads to better mental health of
professionals and improvement in patients' health.

Recent Pilot Research: I conducted with healthcare technology
professionals (N=10) and healthcare providers (N=10) reinforces
these concepts. The results showed exceptionally high
engagement, with 100% of professionals reporting that their work
felt meaningful and 90% describing themselves as inspired and
motivated. While emotional exhaustion was present in some
cases (60% reported occasional fatigue), levels of
depersonalisation remained strikingly low, and all participants
reported strong personal accomplishment. Importantly, 100%
agreed that meaning and purpose directly improved the quality of
healthcare technology, with 40% noting substantial improvements

in both product quality and adoption. Healthcare providers echoed this, with 90% emphasising that professionals' sense of meaning is "extremely important" for successful digital health adoption. These findings provide early empirical support for the arguments in this chapter, demonstrating how positive psychology principles, particularly meaning and purpose, can tangibly enhance both healthcare technology professionals (developer, designer, QA lead etc.) well-being and user facing outcomes in healthcare systems

References:

1. https://linkinghub.elsevier.com/retrieve/pii/S1532046411001328
2. Alawiye, T.R., 2024. The Impact of Digital Technology on Healthcare Delivery and Patient Outcomes. E-Health Telecommun. Syst. Netw. 13, 13–22. https://doi.org/10.4236/etsn.2024.132002
3. Carayon, P., Hoonakker, P., 2019. Human Factors and Usability for Health Information Technology: Old and New Challenges. Yearb. Med. Inform. 28, 071–077. https://doi.org/10.1055/s-0039-1677907
4. Csikszentmihalyi, M., 2002. Flow: the classic work on how to achieve happiness, Rev. and updated ed. ed. Rider, London.
5. Evans, R.S., 2016. Electronic Health Records: Then, Now, and in the Future. Yearb. Med. Inform. Suppl 1, S48-61. https://doi.org/10.15265/IYS-2016-s006
6. Edo, O.C., Ang, D., Etu, E.-E., Tenebe, I., Edo, S., Diekola, O.A., 2023. Why do healthcare workers adopt digital health technologies - A cross-sectional study integrating the TAM and UTAUT model in a developing economy. Int. J. Inf. Manag. Data Insights 3, 100186. https://doi.org/10.1016/j.jjimei.2023.100186

7. Gomes Chaves, B., Briand, C., Bouabida, K., 2021. Innovation in Healthcare Organizations: Concepts and Challenges to Consider. Int. J. Health Res. Innov. 1–14. https://doi.org/10.47260/ijhri/911
8. Graziotin, D., Fagerholm, F., Wang, X., Abrahamsson, P., 2018. What happens when software developers are (un)happy. J. Syst. Softw. 140, 32–47. https://doi.org/10.1016/j.jss.2018.02.041
9. Yablonski, J. (2024). *Laws of UX: Using psychology to design better products & services* [Digital eTextbook edition]. O'Reilly Media
10. Seligman, M. E. P. (2011). *Flourish: A visionary new understanding of happiness and well-bei*

Chapter 10: Customer Journey Maps

Customer Journey Maps (CJM):

Definition - Customer journey maps in healthcare information systems are visual tools that illustrate the step-by-step experience of patients, providers, or other stakeholders as they interact with digital health platforms. They help identify pain points, needs, and emotions at each stage of the healthcare process, from appointment booking to follow-up care. By mapping these experiences, healthcare organizations can design more patient-centred systems that improve usability, satisfaction, and health outcomes. Such mapping is increasingly used in digital health transformation to align technology with patient expectations and care delivery goals

1. Customers, for instance, care intensely about their own needs and desires but they don't generally know or care as much about how companies are organised.
2. Employees also have their individual frames of reference; which often includes a deeper understanding of products, company organisation, and subject matter than do customers.

    a. The perspective of employees is also shaped by the culture of an organisation, the structure and silos created within the organisation, given all those influences on the human psyche, it's hard for any individual to break out from their own perspective.
3. In Self-referential design, we make decisions that satisfy our needs. That's the problem that companies need to avoid.

4. Customers very often have substantially different needs than the employees who are making decisions about how to satisfy them.
5. Customers have their own needs and perspectives. Once we recognize this situation, we can overcome the natural tendency of self-centeredness
6. In addition to not recognizing that we may be interacting with customers many times along a single journey, we also miss opportunities to satisfy customers in other areas along their journey.

   a.   Consider a customer looking to obtain a specific module in the Health information system related to clinical prescribing. A feature that allows the physician to :

   i. Prescribe medicines
   ii. A feature to prescribe either by brand or generic name

7. Why don't we also offer provisions to : (Clinician's journey)

   a.   Check the availability of the medicines within the hospital inventory if the HIS is being developed for a large hospital facility

   b.   Options to prescribe medications according to the patient's medical conditions. For example if the patient is pregnant, suitable alerts to show that specific drugs can or cannot be prescribed for this patient

   c.   Facility to prescribe not only normal medications like paracetamol, iBrufein but also oncology drugs, intravenous fluids for inpatients.

   d.   A clinical calculator facility, for example to calculate BMI of the patient just for reference while prescribing drugs.

   e.   An option to prescribe alternate drugs in case the required brand or generic is not in stock.

8. CJMs are valuable because they help identify how a customer views an organisation by putting the interactions with a company in the context of the customer's broader activities, goals and objectives.

Patient Journeys: In Patient management portal, apart from providing a provision for the patient to view and rescheduling appointments, lab reports etc. features such as:

Updates on latest inventions in their field of disease. For example if the patient is diabetic then specific newsletters on inventions of new drugs to combat diabetes, change in lifestyle etc.

Option for the patient to upload images/files to interact with the physician.

My understanding:

A customer's primary requirement often depends on the fulfilment of certain prerequisites that must be addressed before the main need can be effectively executed. Without these foundational elements, the customer's core requirement may remain unmet. Furthermore, there may be additional provisions or supportive facilities that, while not essential to the main requirement, can enhance the overall service or product delivery. Incorporating these elements helps ensure that the customer's experience is both comprehensive and satisfactory.

References:

1. Patient journey mapping: emerging methods for understanding and improving patient experiences of health systems and services:
2. https://academic.oup.com/eurjcn/article/23/4/429/7597463
3. Journey Mapping 101:
4. https://www.nngroup.com/articles/journey-mapping-101/
5. Patient journey mapping: what it is, its benefits, and how to do it:
6. https://uxpressia.com/blog/patient-journey-mapping

Chapter 11: Final Thoughts – Designing Healthcare Information Systems (HIS) That Evolve with Care

Health Information Systems (HIS) are essential for healthcare, as they influence each aspect of care delivery, like clinical decision-making and patient engagement. HIS directly impacts safety, efficiency, and patient satisfaction.

Let's reflect on the key concepts of the book, and enable the mind-set required to ensure HIS design remains relevant and effective in the future.

Key Takeaways from This eBook

1. User-Centred Design is Non-Negotiable

The guidelines provided in the book point towards system success, when they are built around the people who use them, such as clinicians, nurses, pharmacists, or administrative staff. Their aim should be to simplify tasks rather than make complications. Continuous research, user engagement and ongoing testing form the foundation for effective design.

2. Consistency Builds Trust

Being consistent ensures success and secures the future. Errors can be reduced with uniform layouts, predictable navigation and standardized terminologies, which also can reduce cognitive effort. HIS should be user-friendly and feel familiar across the modules. It allows the users to work seamlessly without any irritation and confusion.

3. Simplicity is Power

Avoid complexity, as it destroy the efficiency. HIS should present the data that matters the most at the right time. It uses hierarchy and logical grouping and minimises the distractions. Cluttered screens should be avoided as they are the warning signs for potential mistakes rather than a sign of completeness.

4. Error Prevention and Recovery Save Lives

Design should build guardrails against them to prevent mistakes. Users can correct their mistakes with the help of the features like real-time validation, meaningful errors or undo options, without any frustration. These small design mean the difference between safety and harm especially in a clinical environment.

5. Iteration is the Lifeblood of Usability

All designs undergo different processes to eliminate errors. Real-world feedback and usability testing help systems to overcome their weaknesses, enable workflow and regulatory demands. **Agile and Lean UX methodologies** make this possible by embedding adaptability into the development process.

6. Training and Support Ensure Adoption

Even the most intuitive system requires guidance. Robust on boarding, in-app help, and easy-to-access training resources bridge the gap between design and real-world use. When users feel confident, adoption rates rise and resistance falls.

Every intuitive system needs guidance, user support strategies like robust on boarding, in-app help and easy-to-access training resources help to connect design and the real-world use.

Adoption rates rise when users feel confidence, it also helps to minimise the resistance.

The Imperative of Continuous Improvement

Healthcare is a continuous process, new technologies, standards and updated care models emerge with time. An evolving design is an asset, as compared to a static HIS design which is a liability. Developers and healthcare organisations must keep the systems aligned with real-world needs and embrace feedback loops, usability metrics and incremental enhancements.

A Call to Action

For HIS designers, developers, and healthcare leaders, the responsibility is clear:

- **Invest in usability research.** Understand real clinical environments before designing solutions.
- **Adopt iterative development.** Regularly test, refine, and release updates to stay relevant.
- **Champion user empowerment.** Provide tools that **assist rather than overwhelm**, supporting better decisions and safer care.
- **Keep ethics and empathy at the core.** Respect user time, protect patient privacy, and design for accessibility and inclusivity.

Healthcare is too critical for design to be an afterthought. Every screen, button, and workflow should serve the ultimate goal: enabling healthcare professionals to focus on patients, not technology.

Closing Note

The accomplishment of a good design depends on its user-friendly characteristics. Users appreciate it when it works well, but any breach may result in consequences such as waste of time, increased frustration among users. So, the system should be intuitive, adaptive, and relentlessly user-friendly.

HIS does not end with deployment, it marks the beginning. By honouring the principles of usability and embracing continuous improvement, we can create systems that **empower clinicians, safeguard patients, and advance the future of healthcare**.

Glossary:

Term	Explanation
Access Control	A security measure that restricts who can view or use resources in a computing environment, ensuring only authorized individuals can access sensitive data or systems, which helps protect confidentiality, integrity, and availability. https://www.sentinelone.com/cybersecurity-101/cybersecurity/what-is-access-control/
Accessibility (WCAG)	Follow WCAG guidelines, enable screen readers, keyboard navigation, and colour contrast options. https://www.wcag.com/resource/what-is-wcag/
Actionable Information	Information that is readily available, easily interpretable, and immediately actionable for effective decision-making.
Agile Development Methodologies	Project management frameworks that break projects into iterative cycles (sprints), allowing rapid adaptation, continuous user feedback, and continuous improvement. https://asana.com/resources/

	agile-methodology
Alert Fatigue	Too many alerts cause users to ignore important warnings; and should be used sparingly.
Audit Trails	Logs that record user actions such as data access, modifications, or deletions.
Authentication (Login Mechanisms)	Secure login using SSO, smart cards, or biometrics to balance security and practicality.
Breadcrumb Trail	A navigation aid that shows user location and allows return to previous pages easily.
Cognitive Load	Effort required to process information; reduced using progressive disclosure and filtering.
Confidentiality	Ensuring patient data is not disclosed without proper authorisation. https://www.hhs.gov/hipaa/for-professionals/security/laws-regulations/index.html
Consistency (Visual Design)	Uniform colours, fonts, and buttons to reduce user confusion and cognitive effort.
Context-Sensitive Help	Embedded interface assistance like tooltips, inline tutorials, and guidance relevant to users' current

	tasks.
Customer Journey Maps (CJMs)	Visual diagrams outlining user interactions, pain points, emotions, and goals throughout their system experience.
Customisable Views	Allow users to configure dashboards and panels for personalised workflows.
Data Aggregation	Combining data from multiple sources into a single interface for a complete view.
Data Visualisation	Presenting data using charts, graphs, and colour-coded indicators.
Drill-Down Navigation	Allows access to detailed information from summaries for clarity.
EHRs (Electronic Health Records)	Digital systems managing patient health data, integrated with other clinical systems
Error Prevention & Feedback	Systems that detect potential errors in real time and offer clear correction guidance.
Error Recovery	Features that provide undo and reversible actions to correct mistakes easily.
Feedback & Iteration	Continuous usability testing and stakeholder feedback during design.
GUI (Graphical User Interface)	Visual interface supporting user workflows and reducing

	cognitive load.
HIPAA	U.S. law ensuring secure and authorised sharing of health information.
HIS (Health Information Systems)	Systems managing patient data and supporting clinical decision-making.
Information Organisation	Structuring information for quick scanning and prioritisation.
Integrity	Protecting health data from unauthorised alteration or destruction.
Interoperability	Ability of different systems to exchange and use information seamlessly.
Keyboard Shortcuts	Key combinations to speed up common actions in the system.
Loading Indicators	Visual indicators showing system status during processing.
Navigation Hierarchy	Clear structure for organising menus and navigation paths.
Nielsen's Sitemap Research	Findings by the Nielsen Norman Group that sitemaps significantly enhance navigation and usability in large-scale systems https://www.nngroup.com/reports/site-map-usability/

Patient Safety in the digital world	Designing interfaces to minimise user error and ensure safe care.
Privacy	The patient's right to keep medical records confidential.
Progressive Disclosure	Showing essential info first and allowing access to details if needed.
RBAC (Role-Based Access Control)	Restricts data access based on user roles to ensure security.
Responsive Design	Adapts interface for desktop, tablet, and mobile devices.
Security (Healthcare Information Security)	Procedures ensuring secure storage and access of health information.
Sitemap	A system overview that helps users navigate when lost.
Status Mechanisms	Indicators and messages to inform users of system state and errors.
Training (End-User Training)	Hands-on practice required for successful system adoption.
UCD (User-Centred Design)	Design approach focused on user needs and feedback for usability.
Undo Functionality	Feature that allows reversing actions to recover from mistakes.
Usability Testing	Evaluating the system through real user testing and feedback.
Visible Navigation	Navigation elements always visible for quick access.

Visual Hierarchy	Organising interface elements for easy scanning and focus.
WCAG (Accessibility Standard)	Standard guidelines for accessible design to support all users.
Wrong-Patient Error Prevention	Displaying patient identifiers to avoid errors on wrong records.
Swivel-Chair Experience	Switching between systems causing inefficiency, reduce productivity at work and errors; should be avoided. https://blog.sisfirst.com/how-to-avoid-swivel-chair-integration-in-health-it
Availability (CIA Triad)	Ensuring health data is available to authorised users when needed. https://www.fortinet.com/uk/resources/cyberglossary/cia-triad

Definitions:

Clinical Decision Support (CDS) refers to systems that analyse data from various clinical and administrative sources to help healthcare providers make informed clinical decisions. The data can assist in preparing diagnoses or predicting medical events, such as drug interactions. These tools filter information to support clinicians in caring for individual patients.

Clinical Decision Support Systems (CDSS) are tools that provide healthcare professionals with evidence-based information and recommendations for patient care.

Electronic Health Records (EHR) are digital versions of patients' paper charts, containing medical histories, diagnoses, treatment plans, and more. EHRs provide a more detailed record of a patient's medical history and include additional health data, test results, and treatments.

Health Information Exchange (HIE) refers to systems that enable the sharing of patient information across different healthcare providers to improve coordination and continuity of care.

Health Information System (HIS) refers to a system designed to manage healthcare data. This includes systems that collect, store, manage, and transmit a patient's electronic medical record (EMR), a hospital's operational management, or a system supporting healthcare policy decisions.

Health Information Technology (HIT) involves the development and implementation of health information systems to support patient care and healthcare management.

Hospital Management Systems (HMS) are software solutions that support the administrative and operational aspects of hospitals, such as patient scheduling, billing, and inventory management.

Master Patient Index (MPI) connects separate patient records across databases. The index maintains a unique record for each patient registered at a healthcare organisation and links all associated records for that patient. MPIs help reduce duplicate records and minimise inaccurate patient information that can lead to claim denials.

Patient Portals provide patients with secure access to their personal health data, such as appointment information, medications, and laboratory results, via an internet connection. Some patient portals also allow active communication with physicians, prescription refill requests, and appointment scheduling.

Practice Management Software helps healthcare providers manage daily operations, including scheduling and billing. Providers ranging from small practices to large hospitals use these systems to automate many administrative tasks.

Remote Patient Monitoring (RPM) is commonly used in telehealth setups and allows medical sensors to transmit patient data to healthcare professionals. The data supports early detection of medical events requiring intervention and may contribute to population health studies.

Telemedicine Systems are platforms that enable healthcare professionals to diagnose, consult, and treat patients remotely through video calls or other digital communication tools.

References:

1. A mini glossary for Digital Health - https://www.linkedin.com/pulse/mini-glossary-digital-health-healthtechxacademy-yjbjc/
2. Health Information Systems: Technological and Management Perspectives: https://www.ncbi.nlm.nih.gov/books/NBK60

www.ingramcontent.com/pod-product-compliance
Lightning Source LLC
Chambersburg PA
CBHW051258020426
42333CB00026B/3259